D0629138

Conquering
Cancer

Lucien Israël, M.D.

Conquering Cancer

Translated from the French by Joan Pinkham

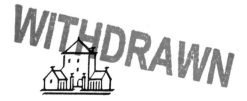

Random House New York

RC
263
.I7813
1978

Copyright © 1978 by Lucien Israël
All rights reserved under International and Pan-American Copyright Conventions.
Published in the United States by Random House, Inc., New York, and simultaneously
in Canada by Random House of Canada Limited, Toronto. Originally published in
France as *Le Cancer aujourd'hui*
by Bernard Grasset, Paris.
Copyright © 1976 by Editions Grasset & Fasquelle

Library of Congress Cataloging in Publication Data

Israel, Lucien,
Conquering cancer,

Translation of Le cancer aujourd'hui.
1. Cancer   1. Title
AC263.I7813   616.9'94
ISBN 0–394–41861–1   78–57382

Manufactured in the United States of America
2 4 6 8 9 7 5 3
First American Edition

To my wife, who did not capitulate to the cancer of Auschwitz

Acknowledgments

I want to thank Nathalie Hottinguer, Raymond Lepoutre, Paul Lochak, and Paul Sachet, whose documentation and friendly cooperation overcame my natural laziness, which would otherwise have prevented me from finishing this book. I also want to express my heartfelt thanks to all my nurses, and especially to my head nurse, Catherine Adonis, who for ten years has been watching over our patients, keeping their spirits up, and smoothing the difficulties in their path.

Foreword

This book hopes to explain—and, if possible, to help reduce—the intolerable discrepancy between the way in which cancer patients are treated today and the way in which they could be treated. In the past ten years there have been real advances, which have considerably increased our power over the disease. In certain cases that were formerly despaired of, it is now possible to attempt a cure; in others, we can substantially prolong life expectancy under conditions that the patients themselves evidently consider acceptable, since they submit to the new treatments when given the choice.

The discrepancy is by no means peculiar to France, or indeed to any country. In all the advanced nations, the attitude of the average doctor lags far behind the progress that has been made by teams in the forefront of clinical research as far as cancer is concerned. A great many doctors are ignorant of the progress or deny it or even oppose it, and many patients are still treated the way they were ten or more years ago. As was so often the case in the nineteenth century, medical opinion today is divided, and each side defends its position with passion. But the kind of controversy that raged in the nineteenth century is no longer acceptable in an age when medicine is becoming more and more scientific and every physician is able to keep himself informed, to learn about results obtained by others, and to modify his own practice accordingly.

I therefore propose to present all the information on cancer that is readily available but that, so far as I know, has not yet been gathered between covers, either for practicing physicians or for the interested public. I don't think it can do any harm to disseminate this information to nonspecialists. There is no reason today to protect men and women from the truth, and in any event, it is not for doctors to arrogate to themselves the right to do so, and safe from questioning or contradiction, to decide by themselves what they will or will not do to help the sick. The various interested parties must have access to everything in the file. The task of providing this is an urgent one because, according to the epidemiologists' latest calculations, one out of every four persons alive today will develop a cancer. At the same time, medicine is making such rapid strides that the possibilities of treatment change from one year to the next.

The reader must not imagine that this book contains unpublished secrets or personal remedies. On the contrary, part of my purpose is to expose charlatans of every type, men who profit from despair and hold back progress by dissuading countless victims of cancer from seeking real help. I want to set forth the latest theoretical and practical results that have been obtained by the international scientific community and that are available to everyone. I have the privilege of being one of the few Europeans admitted to membership in an American cooperative group working under the aegis of the National Cancer Institute of the United States, and of having been given responsibility for some of its clinical studies. Belonging also to the European Organization for Research on the Treatment of Cancer and chairing its section on lung cancer, I have been in a position to be involved in a number of ways with many of the important advances made by a truly fascinating group of people, to whose scientific rigor and daring I here pay tribute.

It is true that both the prime causes of cancer and its innermost mechanisms are still the subject of speculation. And there are many distinguished thinkers who believe that our accomplishments as practicing physicians—as engineers, so to speak—will remain illusory until the molecular biologists have brought those causes and mechanisms to light. I am among those who take vigorous exception to this view. If, today, one little leukemia sufferer out of three has a good chance of being cured, whereas fifteen years ago his or her life expectancy never exceeded three months, the credit goes not to the achievements of molecular biology but to the obstinate, patient efforts of the therapists, among whom members of the French school, headed by Jean Bernard and Georges Mathé, have played a decisive role. The therapists have had to combine the most advanced techniques with a judicious empiricism. They have had to invent a whole methodology of clinical trials and experimental chemotherapy, to develop the fields of cell kinetics and radiobiology, and to perfect many technologies, such as that of sterile environments, for example. It is interesting to note that the oncologists—cancer specialists—have contributed much more to general immunology than the specialists in basic immunology have so far contributed to oncology.

I do not mean to deny the importance of the basic sciences and pure theoretical research. But if in recent years we had depended on them to improve the treatment of cancer, we would not have advanced for practical purposes beyond the results obtained in 1945. In this book I show what important progress has been made since then by clinicians and by the experimenters who work side by side with them, seeking answers to questions that the partisans of basic research consider trivial. I hope that the officials who are responsible for the economics of research will have an opportunity to read these lines and to reflect upon them—and that they may be moved to consult the interested parties before they draw up their overall plans.

But why should anyone believe what I am saying? How is it conceivable that advances in treatment, if they are real, are not immediately incorporated into the practice of every physician? Is it not a kind of paranoid obstinacy to insist that doctors could do better, much better, and yet do not? Of course I intend to answer these questions and to examine the reasons for the discrepancy—a tragic discrepancy, in my opinion—between the possibilities and the reality. I don't expect to persuade everyone to accept my conclusions: naturally, those who are guilty of what I call ignorance—or worse, of a refusal to learn—have to justify their attitude. In this connection, I should like to recall my experiences as a student.

In 1947–48, I witnessed the stupefaction and skepticism of my elders when it became apparent that streptomycin could cure tubercular meningitis and that penicillin eliminated syphilis in a matter of days. In the first instance, when a well-informed practitioner presented a group of cured patients to a very respectable medical society, a specialist of the time didn't hesitate to call the presentation a hoax. As for syphilis, it was not a disease to be treated but a sin to be expiated by twenty years of injections of bismuth, arsenic, and mercury. It was shocking to think that it could be cured in a week. When the young doctors in hospitals, relying on the work of American clinicians and on their own clinical and biological observations, offered proof of that fact, they were greeted with insults and disbelief.

Today, within the medical establishment, skepticism is still considered in good taste, while enthusiasm and innovation are severely frowned upon. This attitude is more prevalent in the field of cancer than in any other, and it is easy to see its connection with the supernatural. It is the doctors as much as the public who are responsible for making cancer a thing of the devil. The irrational, driven from every hiding place, must hold some ground, after all. The same physician who sends a patient with severe coronary thrombosis to an intensive-care unit, or who recommends a kidney transplant to a patient whose chances are slim, takes it upon himself to advise the family to abstain from treatment of an advanced cancer, or even a localized one. This, in defiance of modern medical knowledge, of which either he is ignorant or he denies, and of the interests of his patient, whom he does not consult. There must be a reason for this, and I want to go into that question in greater detail at the end of this book.

I also want to show how the small international community of oncologists makes progress, how it draws up strategies, tests them, and little by little optimizes its results. The term "optimization," which comes from cybernetics, is one I want to emphasize: it stands for the process by which the human mind, advancing into the unknown, first reduces difficulties and then overcomes them. It stands for the process by which, since the beginning of scientific medicine and especially since the spirit of dogmatism was abandoned, physicians have steadily improved the art of curing the sick.

I don't regard empiricism as a failing. If biology lags behind physics, it is because its subject matter is more complex. If human medicine is more disappointing than experimental biology, it is because it deals with the whole person, including the brain, which is one of the most complex structures in the known universe. If oncologists make slower progress than orthopedists, it is because cancer is a disease affecting the most subtle, most fundamental mechanisms of life. (In an increasing order of complexity, we would come to human societies, which no doubt is why political discourse is still so far from being scientific.) But oncologists do make progress nonetheless, and if medical knowledge doubles every five years—actually, it is increasing even faster—it is unimaginable that the study of cancer alone has failed to benefit from the explosion.

I began my work with cancer some ten years ago. Since that time everything has changed, including, above all, the patient's life expectancy, no matter what sort of tumor he has or how far it has developed. The public should know this, and doctors should know it too, despite those who—for lack of information or for, shall we say, more complicated reasons—prefer inertia to forward movement.

For the benefit of those who wish to form an opinion about the controversy over cancer treatment, I set forth the facts that have been established, the problems that have been encountered, the methodologies that have been developed to solve those problems, and the material and psychological obstacles to progress in research. I describe the new weapons forged by oncologists, the results that have been achieved, and those that we can expect in the near future. I conclude by analyzing the causes of the resistance to using such tools that we encounter, and possible ways to overcome this resistance. I ask those of my patients who recognize themselves in my examples to pardon me. They know, even if I have not always said it in so many words, that ours is a common struggle; and I know not only how courageous they are but, in many cases, how altruistic.

I am well aware that I belong to that privileged category of men who are paid to do precisely what is most interesting to them on earth. In the course of my studies, and especially during my internship, I fell in love with the medical profession, and I have no hesitation in saying that I hold it to be one of the noblest, for its purpose is to protect and defend one of the most precious possessions of human beings: their health and the health of their loved ones. The "image" of the doctor today is changing and deteriorating in ways that I do not wish to discuss here. Nevertheless, I am deeply touched, time and again, by the trust that is placed in us in very difficult situations, a trust that is revealed in attitudes, letters, words, silences. In this book, at the risk of starting arguments that are always disagreeable in some ways, I am paying a debt. If society invests us, even reluctantly, with a degree of power over its members, we owe it to society to set forth the facts and to speak the truth.

I also want to explain why, although I was trained in the treatment of pulmonary disorders, I became increasingly involved in oncology, despite the academic traditions in France which—contrary to public statements on the subject—strongly discourage any attempt at interdisciplinary work. I have not renounced my first specialty. It gives me new approaches to one of the central problems of cancer: the mechanisms by which the organism in general and the lungs in particular defend themselves against tumors. I am studying these mechanisms at present. In a world invaded by air pollutants, such research is absolutely essential. But the medical profession does not like to have one of its members carve out a new domain that cuts across two existing specialties. Until the new discipline finally wins acceptance, anyone who practices it is likely to be accused by both sides of being an amateur—and I am deliberately using a euphemism.

Oncologists must remember that they have no legal existence in France. Incredible as it may seem, since we are talking about the disease whose frequency is second only to that of arteriosclerosis and associated cardiovascular disorders, oncology is not a recognized specialty. It is not one of the required courses in medical schools, and with a few rather unconvincing exceptions, it is not practiced in public hospitals and university hospitals. If there are oncologists, they train themselves and co-opt or excommunicate each other the way general practitioners did during the Revolution. That is another reason why this branch of medicine lags behind others, as I mentioned above, and another subject for reflection.

The existing medical structures fall far short of the needs, and this is not because material means are lacking or because the government vetoes change. Rather, it is the particular rigidity of the medical profession and its complex interplay of habits, rivalries, and prestigious positions that are the basic obstacles to progress. Will we, in this domain as in a hundred others, prove ourselves collectively capable of achieving a true liberalism, a dispassionate empiricism that will enable us to test in practice potential remedies for the ills we suffer, or are we doomed to alternate between periods of revolutionary upheaval and periods of mental sclerosis induced by a hidebound, centralized hierarchical establishment? While I was writing this book, I continually asked myself why it is that what should happen does not happen, why glaring faults are not corrected. I firmly resisted all temptation to identify a particular "enemy," because I think it is obvious that such a temptation arises from an ideological prejudice—that is, from a neurotic personality—and has nothing to do with the spirit of scientific inquiry. The practice of my profession has taught me that empiricism is the only honest and also the only operational attitude, for someone who is trying to understand and improve the world around him.

Contents

Part One

❈❈❈

1

❀❀❀

Misconceptions About Cancer

Oncology—the study and treatment of cancer—is a medical specialty that was recognized in the United States only five years ago. In many countries it still does not exist. Most doctors who call themselves oncologists have conferred the title on themselves. Some of them are physicians who came to oncology through hematology, a specialty in which they learned to treat leukemias and lymphomas and to handle drugs that were to prove effective on solid tumors as well. Others were trained as radiologists and consider themselves best qualified to treat cancers and to give direction to clinical research. Still others are surgeons specializing in the removal of malignant tumors.

My own background, as I have said, was in pulmonary disorders. In 1964, when I was associate professor of pulmonary medicine, I became interested in lung cancers. When patients were not operable, they were left to the lung specialists, who treated them without having even a rudimentary understanding of cancer. With the guidance and encouragement of the head of the department, Etienne Bernard, who was doing so much to combat tuberculosis (still a terrible scourge at the time), I began to study, to travel, to try different treatments for the patients who were abandoned to us. Since the lung is one of the organs in which metastases are most likely to appear, I found myself treating pulmonary metastases from breast cancers, bone cancers, cancers of the colon, and so forth. And I realized very soon that I would have to educate myself about chemotherapy, immunology, cell kinetics, and even radiobiology and statistics.

The diversity in the background of oncologists is partly responsible for the controversies that rage in this field, the rivalries and struggles for control of the specialty. It also explains the incredible fact that the treatment strategy drawn up for a given patient is most likely to be determined not by the patient's pathological condition but by the orientation of the doctor he or she consults first. The nature of the treatment will almost certainly depend on whether that doctor was trained as a surgeon, a radiotherapist, or a medical oncologist.

Even worse, there are not nearly enough oncologists in the world today (this is especially true in France), which means that many patients are treated from beginning to end by a specialist in the organ in which the tumor occurs, although he may have no knowledge whatever of cancer—which will not prevent him from having firm opinions on the subject.

Nevertheless, it is in these circumstances that doctors are developing the great innovations in treatment, chemotherapy and immunotherapy, new methods that are only beginning to show their worth, methods that are at last designed to combat not only the visible tumor but also the invisible, disseminated disease that the tumor so often represents. The progress already achieved by these innovations is unfortunately denied by many doctors, whose advice to cancer patients is based either on total ignorance of the new treatments or on solid prejudice against them.

For a long time I hoped that the normal diffusion of knowledge in medical circles would be enough to bring present practice up to the level of present needs and present possibilities. But many examples of resistance to innovations in treatment—conscious or unconscious, organized or diffused—have convinced me that the only way to bring about change is to have an open debate among doctors, public-health administrators, government officials, and patients (past, present, and potential). And in order to have rational debate, it is essential to demystify cancer, not only for the public but also for the medical profession. That is not an easy task—and the technical difficulties are not necessarily the hardest—but we have no choice. First, let us try to clear up some misconceptions.

Optimism about surgery: the "five-year cure"

Statements issued to the public imply that the first radical treatment applied to a tumor—be it surgical excision, radiotherapy, or a combination of the two—cures one to two patients out of three. This makes it appear that medical treatment is only supplementary and that the way to raise the percentage of cures is through earlier detection—which will bring to the surgeon or radiotherapist cases of more recent origin —rather than through advances in medical treatment. This deduction is, however, incorrect.

The fact that a patient survives for five years after an operation does not imply that he is cured. Precise statistics published by a few centers show that, because of metastases, mortality from cancer persists beyond ten years, and sometimes beyond fifteen years. Accordingly, while the surgeon whose patient has passed the five-year mark has every right to be pleased, he cannot be completely easy in his mind and is not entitled to dissuade a similar patient from undertaking longer-range treatment. The limit of five years was chosen because the number of recurrences drops off between five and fifteen years. But here the statistics are deceptive: the number of recurrences drops after five years only because the total number of survivors has dropped significantly by then and continues to do so. In reality, the curves show that between one month and ten years, the rate of death remains constant. In other words, the *rate* at which recurrences appear remains the same, though in a steadily reduced population. So while there are indeed cases that are cured by the initial treatment, they are, unfortunately, less numerous than the statistics proclaim.

These statistics, moreover, relate to the period of survival between the operation or radiotherapy and the death of the patient. They do not relate to the free interval between the initial treatment and a recurrence of the disease. Since, fortunately, patients can have a recurrence and still survive, the two periods of time are not identical. But most authors do not trouble to distinguish between them when reporting their results, and the duration of "apparent cure" is therefore shorter than most studies indicate.

In the majority of cancers, when we examine a patient between one and ten years after the intervention, it is impossible to determine whether or not he is cured—that is, whether or not he harbors malignant cells, cells which, while their presence is not revealed by any symptom, may cause a severe recurrence at some future time. Perhaps we will one day have precise tests, biological "markers" that can be measured so exactly that if they are absent after a given period of time, we can state that the patient is cured. Only a short while ago, patients with Hodgkin's disease who had lived beyond fifteen years were considered cured. But recent studies have raised disturbing doubts: it seems that when autopsies were performed on certain of these patients after accidental death, they were found to have harbored perfectly identifiable uncured lesions. Did this mean that there had been a regular process of regrowth starting from the "last cell" left intact by the treatment, or were these lesions that were temporarily quiescent but capable of resuming their evolution someday?

I shall answer this question later. For the time being, all we need to understand is this: at present there is no way of being absolutely certain that an individual case of cancer is cured. While it is true that the chances of cure increase with the passage of time, we must admit, if we are scrupulous, that "cure" can be defined only statistically. If, for example, out of a hundred patients who have had lung operations, twenty-five survive three years later, and if from that time on, their mortality curve is parallel to that of a population of the same age and characteristics without cancer, then those twenty-five were cured. This statistical fact is of fundamental importance for the therapist evaluating successive advances, but it is very inadequate for the patient and his doctor. Fixing a five-year limit for purposes of evaluation is convenient, but it leads the medical profession to overestimate the percentages of cure and hence to underestimate the possible importance of postoperative treatment in a total strategy for improving results.

It is in the name of this groundless optimism—groundless because not all the operated-upon patients who reach the five-year point are free from recurrences, and those who are can't be sure that they will remain so—that many physicians reject modern postoperative treatments, because they might "impair the quality of life" of patients who may be cured. There is a double misconception here: first, these treatments have become infinitely less offensive than they were only five years ago, and at the same time more effective; second, and more important, it is not so much the patient's quality of life that is impaired as the doctor's intellectual comfort. Experience proves that when the patient who has undergone an operation knows what is at stake, he always accepts the possible disadvantages of further treatment. Two of my patients have chosen to abstain, as against hundreds who have agreed to prolonged treatment. And when, after two years of a therapy that I consider sufficient, I want to stop, while there are some patients who rejoice, there are others who say to me, "Are you sure it's wise? Wouldn't it be better to go on for another few months?" The advocates of abstention from treatment have a final argument: they declare that the measures I am talking about are ineffective or even harmful. That is why later on in this book I shall give the statistics of the international groups who practice these procedures.

I must add that, setting aside the small percentage of mortality that is inevitable in any major surgery, a great many cases are discovered too late to benefit from surgical treatment. While it is true that in cancers affecting external organs, such as the breast, radical surgery can be performed in 90 to 100 percent of the cases, it is also true that in cancers of the deep organs, such as the lungs, esophagus, or pancreas, the situation is just the opposite.

Therefore, we must not only take exception to the use of the term "five-year cure," but remember that five-year survival, however dubious that parameter may be, is calculated on the basis of only a part of the total number of cases—that is to say, those that can be treated by surgery.

Pessimism about medicine: "Let them die in peace!"

If not everyone is cured by radical treatment, it is because there are two other categories of patients: those in whom the disease when first discovered is already too disseminated to permit curative surgery or radiotherapy, and those who have recurrences after such treatment. Most consultants, both physicians and surgeons, who are called upon to give an opinion on medical treatment for such patients reject it on the grounds that it is ineffective and toxic. But there are many—including me—who think that this is no longer true in many cases, and that those who deny a patient a treatment that might be of benefit assume a heavy responsibility.

It is obvious to all clinicians that there are certain cases that are evolving so rapidly, in which the disease has become so disseminated and invasive and the physiological equilibrium so precarious, that the patient cannot be successfully treated by any means at our disposal. The most enthusiastic and unthinking therapist knows that even if an improvement could be obtained, it would be for only a few weeks and at the cost of very uncomfortable treatments that would add to the patient's distress. I am opposed to a relentless insistence on treatment in such situations, and I tell the family so. With their complicity, we organize a system of surveillance and minimal care designed primarily to make the patient more comfortable but also to spare him the anguish of being abandoned.

Here lies the real problem today: in more and more cases, it is no longer a choice between leaving the patient in peace (with morphine) and insisting, irresponsibly and sadistically, on treating him. Rather, it is a choice between leaving him in peace—that is, leaving him to die —and obtaining for him a prolonged period of survival under conditions that he finds acceptable. Thanks to the treatments and strategies that are described and discussed in this book, and which hundreds of oncologists are working to improve, it is often possible to control the proliferation of a tumor for a long time, even in cases that most doctors still consider hopeless. The fact that we can achieve this control, by combining radiotherapy and chemotherapy for example, means that certain cancers become chronic diseases, their evolution sometimes being contained for years by treatments, which the patients demand and which are no less tolerable than those administered to persons with kidney transplants. Many of our patients who are in this situation know it. They know that to survive today may mean to survive until the next important discovery. They also have the joy of being with their loved ones, of seeing their children or grandchildren grow up. Some of them —my apologies to those who say we poison our patients—continue to work. I don't even rule out the possibility that certain of them who were considered incurable in the beginning may indeed be cured, contrary to all expectation.

In 1971, a young man of twenty-two was referred to us at Lariboisière Hospital. After a year of various treatments elsewhere, he was bedridden and screaming with pain despite analgesics. He had disseminated tumors of embryonic origin. He knew it. Wonder of wonders, his radiotherapist, who lived in a town near Paris, did not admit defeat and asked us for advice. We suggested a combination of chemotherapy and immunotherapy, including, among others, drugs that our friends at the U.S. National Cancer Institute send us in generous quantities free of charge. We were able to obtain a remission, which the radiotherapist completed. The young man went back to work part time, had a relapse, other remissions. As I write these lines, he is not in pain. He is fighting courageously. He is not cured, but he's grateful to us for not having capitulated and for having fought side by side with him for four and a half years. I do not believe he can be cured. Should I refuse to go on treating him?

Eight years ago, at a time when our techniques were less effective than they are today, I received a posthumous letter. Its author had died a few days before, after struggling for two and a half years against a disseminated cancer of the lung. He had always known the diagnosis and the prognosis, he said, and he thanked me for the unlooked-for reprieve that had enabled him to complete his children's education. During those two and a half years, we had seen each other twice a month for medical treatments, and it had sometimes been necessary to hospitalize him. He had accepted everything and lived with full knowledge of the truth, a fact of which I had been unaware.

Two years ago I saw for the first time a very young woman who had diffuse metastases throughout the skeleton from an acute breast cancer that had been operated on shortly before. An invalid, she preferred to be brought to the weekly treatment sessions rather than to be hospitalized. We had never yet succeeded in controlling so serious a process, but our experience with a few cases that had been less extensive encouraged us to attempt a real chemotherapy and not merely make some magic passes with ineffective doses. For a long time the evolution of the disease remained uncertain, but the pains receded and the patient's general condition slowly improved. She has since resumed her activities, and the various X-rays and isotopic examinations show an improvement that we dared not hope for, although it is still incomplete. We are continuing.

Another woman in a similar situation has just finished three years of treatment, and all her examinations show her to be cured. From beginning to end, she struggled against me, demanding that I reduce the frequency of the inconvenient chemotherapy sessions, threatening to stop all treatment. But that was her way of expressing aggression. She stuck it out and has no regrets.

Another case: Fifteen metastases in each of the two lungs, in a man of thirty-five. After six weeks of a new treatment developed on the basis of data from an American colleague in Buffalo, only two remain, and the patient, who had been hospitalized, has returned home and will continue his treatment in our ambulatory unit for chemotherapy and immunotherapy. I can't tell what the long-range course of the disease will be. But in bringing him to us, his wife defied the advice of two physicians.

Just recently, one of my colleagues entrusted to me a man of forty-five who had been operated on several years earlier for a cancer of the parotid gland. Pulmonary metastases that were growing very slowly made it hard for him to breathe. He was all the more determined to seek help because he knew his diagnosis. A distinguished lung specialist had advised him against consulting an oncologist and had written to the man's doctor, saying "What's the use?" The patient had to convince his doctor that he understood the situation, was ready to try anything, and wanted other opinions. I gave him mine: with appropriate treatment, he could hope not for cure but for prolonged stabilization, a respite I judged would last from one to four years. He immediately began treatment. He is still perfectly fit and goes to work every day. He knows, as I do, that in four years there may be many changes in the treatment of cancer. He wants to try his luck. He earnestly requests the "overzealous insistence on treatment" that some would virtuously wish to spare him.

These examples have been chosen from hundreds. Of course there are cases in which we fail, either immediately or after a few weeks or months of hope. But the cases in which we do have some success show that certain advanced cancers, despite their size and gravity, are no longer necessarily beyond the reach of modern therapeutic resources, and that a physician no longer has the right to declare it's useless to do anything until he has tried a coherent course of treatment. The percentage of cases of prolonged control of the disease is increasing slowly but surely. One rule should be firmly established: do not prolong a treatment that proves ineffective. But effectiveness can be determined quickly, in a very few weeks. To refuse to try a treatment on the ground that it may produce some unwanted side effects, when it might prove effective for a long period of time, is an act so mindless and irresponsible that it should be punishable by law—unless the decision corresponds to the categorical wishes of the patient. Besides, as we shall see when we consider the whole question of chemotherapy, oncologists have developed objective criteria for evaluating palliative treatments, criteria on which there is general agreement. The chief danger today, therefore, is not that patients will receive ineffective treatment. It is that a potentially effective treatment may be withheld from them in the name of a "charity" that is especially open to question because it is not the patients themselves who make the choice.

When we observe the slow optimization of the results obtained in cases of disseminated cancers, we find once again the fundamental difference between the basic scientist and the practicing physician. The former, in his search for the ultimate mechanisms of the disease, is trying to find the miracle pill we are all praying for; the latter, fighting in the front lines, as it were, and taking advantage of the smallest shreds of partial knowledge, tries to relieve suffering, to prolong life, to help nature—and is sometimes able to cure. If oncologists the world over had taken the advice that is often offered them and waited until the molecular biologists had given them the ultimate weapon, an incalculable number of patients now alive and cured or "controlled" would be dead. And we would not have the knowledge that makes it possible for us to look forward to promising developments in the near future, because that knowledge was acquired in the field, under the pressure of necessity, by those hard-working journeymen known as medical practitioners, among whom I am proud to be numbered.

The medical profession is racked with controversy. This is a comforting spectacle when we remember the resistance to change that has characterized the past decades. But now we must gain time—that is, lives. We can no longer deny patients the benefit of certain treatments, either because we are sure they will recover without them, or because we are sure they will die despite them. There is much to be done—and it can be done—to raise the percentage of curable cancer cases, starting today. There is even more to be done—and it, too, can be done—to prolong the lives of those who cannot yet be cured.

2

❊❊❊

What Cancer Is

Cancers have been recognized since ancient times, but we still don't know much about what causes them, what their mechanism is, or how they function. When I was a student, a few viruses had been identified in leukemias in chickens; certain tumors—experimental cancers—had been induced in rats by tars or various chemical agents and by hormones. But the cell had scarcely been studied, the little organoids of which it is composed hadn't all been identified, the biochemical functioning of its hereditary transmission wasn't known. Consequently, we had not the least idea of the way in which cancer modified this normal functioning.

We know a little more about these things now, but still not enough to be able to describe cancer the way we describe an infection, identifying precisely its cause, the way in which it sets in motion the visible or invisible changes that are the disease, and the chain of consequences that result, in space and time, biochemically and structurally. We have therefore to give an external description of cancer and to make hypotheses, on the basis of what is known, about the process of canceration. We must begin by describing the anomalies of the cell, for it is in the cell—in the component common to all organs, that functional unit of life which is still so mysterious—that cancer is born.

A disease of the cell

The cancer cell is a profoundly abnormal cell, as was observed more than a century ago by means of an optical microscope with only modest magnifying power. A cancer cell's morphology is grossly different from that of a healthy cell. Its nucleus is larger and irregular, and there is practically no cell organoid that does not show, by some modification of form, size, or number, the mark of canceration. The old anatomist-pathologists often used the term "monstrous" to describe the cancer cell. It would be surprising if such gross modifications in form were not accompanied by subtler modifications in the physiology, biochemistry, and heredity of these individual cells.

One characteristic of the cancer cell is striking to everyone and of great importance to specialists: when a cancer cell comes into contact with another cell, it continues to proliferate, while two healthy cells that touch each other ordinarily do not. This contact inhibition, which by means of a signal whose nature is not yet understood provides "birth control" within a population of cells, is a curious property of normal cells. In a cancer, the signal is either not emitted or not received. The membrane surrounding each cell—which is not merely a sac but a very complex organ with many different functions—has lost the capacity to obey this regulating order from a higher level. There are many other anomalies—peculiarities of mobility, respiration, and so on—in the way a cancer cell functions. One of these peculiarities has to do with differentiation. Normal tissue almost always contains "stem" cells—that is, undifferentiated cells whose reproductive power remains intact, which are often capable of producing a variety of different specialized cells. If some of the cells of which a tissue is composed are destroyed and eliminated, either by accidental injury or by a regular phenomenon, stem cells start to proliferate. In a few generations (each lasting from several hours to several days), their descendants undergo a progressive differentiation. which finally results in cells totally and exclusively adapted to a single function, that of the organ of which they are a part.

Cancer cells, on the contrary, are not differentiated, or they are differentiated insufficiently or wrongly: not differentiated, when, as is often the case, the tumor has a proliferating core that is composed of stem cells; insufficiently differentiated, in most cases, because cells that are only partially differentiated, with no rhyme or reason, do not respond to regulating signals, of humoral origin for example; wrongly differentiated, because it often happens that a cancer cell in the lung inappropriately secretes hormones of the adrenal glands, or of the parathyroid, or of the posterior part of the pituitary. In this sense, one might say that cancer is a disease of the differentiation of cells. But one might equally well say that it is a disease of the cell's respiratory or reproductive functions.

In a cancer, the reproduction of cells takes place in a highly abnormal fashion. It has long been known that, contrary to what occurs in healthy cells, when cancer cells divide, the number of chromosomes varies from one cell to another within the same tumor. The variations in time and space can be very great; the daughter cells do not necessarily contain an identical number of chromosomes. There are many other visible anomalies, which are a nightmare for the specialists.

All these abnormalities of morphology and functioning necessarily have corresponding biochemical abnormalities. There are differences— some known, others suspected, many doubtless unknown—between cancer cells and normal cells in the structure, distribution, and functioning of their enzymatic machinery, as well as in their consumption and transportation of energy and their mechanisms for storing it. These differences are still too subtle to be exploited simply and precisely in therapy, but an exploration and analysis of them should lead to progress in the not too distant future.

Cancer is also a disease of cell heredity, which is a major disorder. The differences in the structure and functioning of the enzymes, the membrane, the various organoids, are coded by a hereditary material that is different from normal material. The deoxyribonucleic acid (DNA) of the nucleus, which stores and carries all the information that enables daughter cells to reproduce the mother identically, is not the same in the cancer cell. It is, understandably, especially difficult to measure this difference, but in certain cases it has been possible to show that such a difference does indeed exist, that some of the information represented in the DNA molecule is added and some is missing. In other words, cancer cells are, strictly speaking, mutant cells. The causes, known or suspected, of these mutations will be examined later.

For the time being, let us accept the idea of mutation, which sheds light on everything I've said so far, and go back to the question of the inappropriate secretion of hormones or other substances.

All the cells in an organism are the descendants of a single cell—that is, the egg produced by the fertilization of an ovum by a spermatozoon. Therefore, they all have exactly the same general program, and it is the process of differentiation that assigns them a single special function by "repressing" the expression of other functions. It is a partial "de-repression" that is responsible for the secretion of insulin, or some other hormone, by a lung cell. This "de-repression," a result of canceration, is connected to the way in which the information carried by the DNA is communicated to the operational levels of the cell. Here again the mutation that has made the cell an alien comes into play. The destiny of the cancer cell is not to resemble its sisters or to obey the regulations of a superior order; the cancer cell is a wild and totally asocial individual, programmed to proliferate without restraint, to compete with its neighbors for food, and in the end, to destroy the organism at whose expense it survives. It is probable that not all the cells in a given tumor are viable, and that those that survive are selected by a true short-term Darwinian process. Since useless proliferation is one of the characteristics of cancer tissue, the tumor has an advantage over normal tissue in that it has the time to try one combination after another to find the most "efficient."

We might think of the cell as a factory, a unit of production run entirely by a computer, programmed to choose and establish one particular type of production and equipped with "sensors" capable of regulating the rate of production in accordance with external needs, of selecting the necessary raw materials from the outside environment, and so forth. The cancer cell is a factory whose program is completely out of order, which manufactures useless and harmful products along with its usual products, and which takes no account of external needs, expands and proliferates unnecessarily, and diverts to its own advantage the raw materials useful to its neighbors. In such a situation many would be tempted to bomb the factory that had gone mad. But as we shall see, that is not so simple.

A disease of the tissue

The reader will recall that the proliferation of cancer cells does not obey the regulating signal of contact inhibition. This means that the tissue in which such proliferation is taking place is subject to anarchic growth. If, under certain conditions, we surgically remove part of a rat's liver, the organ grows back, and a signal we do not yet understand stops the growth when the liver regains its original weight and form. In organs that don't reconstitute themselves in this way, the same signal functions during the life of the embryo or at the end of the period of normal growth. The general program of the organism assigns to each of the various tissues a predetermined place, form, and volume. When a cancer appears in an organ, it adopts a certain number of structural and functional characteristics from that organ—more or less of them, as the case may be—but it grows as much as local conditions allow, in defiance of the organism's needs and original program.

This is an important characteristic of cancer tissue, but it is not exclusive to such tissue. There are benign, noncancerous tumors—lipomas or fibromas, for example—that proliferate inappropriately and for no reason. But they remain "encapsulated," separated along their entire periphery from the neighboring healthy tissue, which they compress but do not invade. The borders of the cancer, on the other hand, are blurred or nonexistent. The cancer invades the successive layers of neighboring tissues and adjacent organs one after another, including the walls of the body, the skeleton, and so forth. This is the chief difference, on the local level, between a cancer and healthy tissue or a benign tumor. In particular, it explains the pain experienced in certain cases: the cancer is invading nerve sheaths and compressing and irritating nearby fine nerves, whereas a benign tumor would slowly and delicately push them aside.

What was true for the cancer cell is therefore true for cancer tissue as well. It has lost its function, it defies the laws that assign it a well-defined place in the economy of the organism. It lives its own life, destroying everything around it until key functions are compromised.

Many of the phenomena that occur in cancer tissue are still only suspected or entirely unknown. Among the substances produced by tumors are some that are hormonal in nature and closely resemble secretions which, while inappropriate to the organ in question, would be normal elsewhere. But there are others that are probably entirely "invented" by the cancer. For example, what is the reason for the loss of weight so frequently observed in cancer patients, sometimes when there is only a small, local tumor? What is the reason for the accompanying anemia? Some of these same substances have the effect of protecting the tumor itself against the environment. One of them, recently isolated by American researchers, increases the growth of the small blood vessels, making it possible for the tumor to receive blood—that is, the oxygen and nutritive materials without which it could neither grow nor survive.

To go back to our metaphor of the factory, the different units of production have now joined together. They proliferate, send toxic products to the outside, encroach upon the territory of the units that have remained normal, infiltrate them, compress and destroy them, feed off their substance. The group of crazy units is armed for attack, while the normal units have no means of defense. The factory is not even programmed to respect the structures on which its own survival depends: if it encounters a conduit through which it receives raw materials, or through which the finished products are evacuated, it will obstruct or shatter it, and all activity will cease.

The metastases

Another essential characteristic of cancer tissue is that it does not stay in one place but reproduces itself elsewhere in the organism. When a normal lung or breast cell divides, the two daughter cells remain where they are and serve to renew the tissue from which they came. It is very different with cancer cells. While some remain attached where they are born, others begin to travel. They infiltrate the blood vessels by the thousands and tens of thousands and circulate throughout the organism. Many die on the way, but others stop where they encounter favorable conditions, settle down, reproduce, and colonize the new tissue. What no normal cell is capable of, every cancer cell can do. It grows, regardless of local conditions and the structure of the host tissue, and its descendants reproduce more or less crudely the tissue from which it came. Thus fragments of intestine, bone, or stomach will be found in the lung. This peculiarity, the dissemination of metastases, is fundamental, because it determines the nature of anticancer strategies. It appears very early, during the first few days of a tumor's development. In the short run, our crazy little factories have a method to their madness. They quickly send their offspring out to hide in normal units and to reconstitute little colonies that undertake the same work of proliferation and destruction as the mother colony. From that time on, it is useless to destroy the latter unless one can at the same time identify and destroy the former.

A disease of the entire organism

In the complex, diversified, and hierarchical society that is a living organism, there are certain specialized groups of cells whose function it is to protect the organism against foreign aggression: this is the immunological system, which I want to describe briefly.

When there is an invasion of microbes, for example, they are recognized as alien because of the "antigenic patterns" of the proteins present on the germ walls—that is, because of certain structures that are different from those of all the normal cells of the host and their circulating proteins. A special category of leukocytes, the polymorphonuclear cells, goes to meet the microbes and proliferates in order to phagocytize them—that is, to absorb and destroy them. Another category of leukocytes, the macrophages, is "activated" and does the same thing, but also "prepares" the antigenic patterns in such a form that the information they carry is available to a third series of leukocytes, the B-lymphocytes. These proliferate so as to manufacture antibodies, circulating substances capable of recognizing and neutralizing—or at least attaching themselves to—the particular antigen and that antigen only. Thereafter, B cells with a memory will remain on the alert throughout the life of the organism, ready to start proliferating immediately if the same antigen appears again.

During the "conflict" between the antigens and antibodies, another important factor, of humoral origin, intervenes: the complement, which through the intermediary of the antibody binds itself to the germs and kills them. Another type of antibody binds itself to the

macrophages and enables them to participate in the struggle by phago-
cytizing the structures that carry the antigen. Finally, a fourth category
of leukocytes, the T-lymphocytes, enters the fray. The T-lymphocytes
receive the antigen in an appropriate form through the intermediary
of the macrophages. Some of them kill the foreign microbe cells directly. Others secrete various lymphokines, substances that take part in
the defense through various mechanisms. Still others "help" the
B-lymphocytes increase their secretion of antibodies. Lastly, there are
"suppressive" T-lymphocytes which give the B-lymphocytes the signal
to stop, so as to limit the manufacture of antibodies strictly to the
demand, and which also, under certain circumstances, prevent the
B-lymphocytes from turning against the host's own antigenic patterns.
The respective roles played by the B-lymphocytes and T-lymphocytes
in the immune response are determined both by the genetic characteristics of the individual and by the structure, presentation, and quantity
of the antigens. Transplant immunity is chiefly dependent on T-lymphocytes, microbe immunity on B-lymphocytes.

One point about the "blocking" factors is still controversial. Is it
possible that certain antibodies, attaching themselves in great numbers
to the target cells but not to the complement, shield the foreign cells
from attack by the T-lymphocytes and macrophages? Is this role played
by circulating antigen-antibody complexes? Or is it an excess of antigen
that, attaching itself to the receptors of the lymphocytes and macrophages, blocks their defense functions? Many investigators lean toward
the latter hypothesis, and this is not the place to review their arguments. But I mention the problem in order to point out how some
immune responses might facilitate rather than inhibit the proliferation
of foreign cells.

There is one more essential point to examine. What is the relationship between the immunological system—a system that is present in
nearly all vertebrates and is particularly well developed in mammals—
and cancer?

It is interesting to note that all the research designed to identify
antigens peculiar to cancer cells in spontaneous tumors and in most
experimental tumors that survive by successive transplants yields positive results. In other words, cancer should give rise to victorious immune responses. It does nothing of the kind—if it did, the disease

would not exist. Why? This is a fundamental question. A number of answers, which are not mutually exclusive, have been offered in the past few years. Rough though they are, we can already try to exploit these explanations in treatment, and attempts to do so are very promising.

The first explanation is surprising, as obvious facts sometimes are. The immune mechanism whose operation I have just outlined does not often fail. Since cancer is a particularly frequent phenomenon in the cell, it is possible, and even probable, that our bodies produce several cancers every day, which are relentlessly tracked down and eliminated. But all it takes is one lapse of the system for the tumor to develop and rapidly become ineradicable.

We also know that there are congenital failures of immunity, characterized by repeated infections in early childhood. It is especially significant that in such subjects the risk of cancer is from ten to a hundred times greater than in a normal population of the same age. We might go further and ask if we are sure we have identified all the congenital immunologic disorders, or if it is more likely that we know only the most obvious of them, the ones whose presence is easiest to demonstrate. We can't rule out the possibility that science may in the future analyze more subtle deficiencies, which would account for a large number of cancers. If so, to detect and correct those deficiencies would be an effective preventive measure. Much work needs to be done in this area, but we already have the technology necessary to make a detailed analysis of the immune mechanisms of cancer patients and members of their families. It is to be hoped that a sufficient number of specialists will want to devote themselves to this study, rather than stay in their laboratories waiting for those rare cases that provide new insights.

Continuing the survey of the possible causes for immunologic failure that might make it possible for a cancer to develop, we come to an important and thorny problem: from eighty to a hundred times more cancers appear in persons who have had organ transplants, whose immunologic defenses have had to be artificially lowered, than in a normal population. This underscores the nature of the relations between cancer and immunological status, but two further facts should be noted. First, a hundred times more cancers than in a normal population still represents only a small risk, much smaller than the risk of not carrying out an indispensable transplant. Second, the recipients of transplants who develop cancers don't develop just any tumor, but basically tumors of the immunologic organs themselves and the supporting tissues. This peculiarity has attracted the attention of researchers. Indeed, it may throw light on the immune surveillance mechanism and may even suggest a method of prevention based on it.

Some of the acquired immune deficiencies are caused by infectious diseases, particularly viral diseases such as hepatitis or measles. Others are caused by drugs such as cortisone or by toxic substances such as alcohol. Since cancer is a disease that develops very slowly, we can't rule out the possibility that a cancer that gets its start because of an acquired and lasting immune insufficiency can't be detected until several years later. At present no one knows whether or not it would be useful to test the immunological status of adults on a regular basis and to stimulate or reinforce immunity when it was found wanting. In order for researchers to obtain a conclusive answer, it would be necessary to conduct a study on tens of thousands of voluntary subjects over a period of several years so as to determine whether persons whose spontaneous immunity is lowered are more likely candidates for cancer in the years to follow. It would be an ambitious, difficult, and costly study, but one that might be of primary importance.

In any event, when we test the immunologic capabilities of cancer patients, we often find them diminished, even in patients in whom the tumor has been discovered early and hasn't weakened the organism. But it is also true that a certain number of patients retain their immunologic capabilities intact. How does it happen, then, that they have tumors? One hypothesis is that these tumors are antigenically "weak" —that is, that the organism is deceived by a similarity between the structure of its own proteins and the structure of the tumor's proteins. According to this hypothesis, a cancer with different antigens would be eliminated, but another, more fit for survival, would pass through the net. This would also be the case with cancers having the same transplantation antigens as the host.

There is an entirely different explanation, which also has a great many experimental and clinical arguments in its favor. Cancers—some of them, at any rate—are able to defend themselves against the immune mechanism of the host by secreting substances that hold the macrophages and lymphocytes in check, fend them off, or damage them. Not long ago there was much talk about the work done in this area by the Pasteur Institute and about the interesting research of Fauve and Jacob. Their work completes a series of studies that oncologists all over the world have conducted over the past ten years. All types of immunity may be affected in cancer patients: such patients are often prevented from reacting not only to the specific antigen of their own tumor but also to several different antigens, those of microbes, fungi, or parasites. I myself have shown, however, that in one-third of the subjects, when the tumor was surgically removed, the nonspecific immunity reappeared; and that group of patients thereafter enjoyed a much better prognosis than those whose immunity was not spontaneously restored after the operation. The next step is to try to identify the substances responsible for the weakening of immunity, and then see if we can eliminate or modify them. Along with many other investigators, I am pursuing this line of research, which may one day lead to fortunate results.

We now know that the organs of immunity must be preserved wherever possible. These include the lymph nodes, spleen, thymus, tonsils, and appendix—all of which used to be frequently removed, before we understood their role. In essence, the leukocytes are born in the bone marrow, and it is in these organs that they receive the specialized training that prepares them for action.

One further point: it is generally agreed that one cancer out of a hundred thousand, after it has developed to the point where it is inoperable, will have a spontaneous regression. Such regressions occur most often during severe attacks of infectious diseases accompanied by fever. Many investigators are tempted to think that they are attributable to the stimulation of immunity by the infection. It was this hypothesis that led the American surgeon William B. Coley eighty years ago to try treating cancer with bacterial extracts, an attempt that laid the foundation for certain forms of modern immunotherapy. Rare though they are, these spontaneous regressions are fascinating as models of a therapeutic situation. What nature accomplishes, man can understand, reproduce, and bend to his purpose. That premise is the basis for all biological and medical research.

This discussion of immunity fits in nicely with the metaphor of the factory. Among the normal units of production, there is a mobile police force with an arsenal of highly differentiated weapons that enables it to recognize and destroy "foreign" organisms almost as soon as they are born. Every time a program goes out of order, the factory starts manufacturing new products, which are identified as such, and the police force rushes to the spot.

But the defense can't always be counted upon. The police may be tired or too few in number and may be overwhelmed. They may be deceived by the close similarity between normal products and those manufactured by the units whose program has gone awry. Or those units may have effective anti-police weapons with which they repulse or annihilate the forces of intervention. Lastly, a particularly disturbing phenomenon may occur: the police forces themselves may become cancerous and begin to proliferate wildly. I will say no more about this, because it occurs in diseases of the blood, which are outside my competence.

Cancer and the nervous system

Here I should be brief and say only that no one knows anything about the connections between these two. Many propositions are, however, put forward, as is always the case in areas where the advance of science has not yet penetrated. Many psychiatrists think that not everyone is susceptible to cancer, that there must be a predisposition for the disease. Some think it is a question of personality type. According to them, studies indicate that the typical cancer patient tends to be passive so that his aggression finds only limited expression. Others believe that the predisposition stems from the neurotic history of the patient. Wilhelm Reich even went so far as to place the blame on sexual frustration and repression—quite gratuitously, in light of the evidence. I have nothing against hypotheses, even daring ones—least of all daring ones—provided their authors do not present them as scientific truths, because to do that reflects a totalitarian ideology that claims to have an explanation for everything.

The truth is that we know very little about the relations between cancer and the psyche. But I will say this: on the experimental level it has been shown that in certain strains of rats with a very high incidence of spontaneous leukemia, the frequency of the disease drops abruptly if we place two male rats in each cage instead of one. They fight constantly, bite each other, wound each other, are always on the alert, and something that we do not yet understand happens. On a more general level, I acknowledge that the human psyche can have an effect on a disease like cancer. The fact that evolution has endowed us with so powerful an integrating mechanism is not without consequences. The proposition that a situation of distress can cause a lowering of immunity is by no means either impossible or scientifically shocking. Only, it must be demonstrated first and explained afterward. The fact that once the disease declares itself, a sound emotional balance can be an additional asset is confirmed every day—within certain limits. The hypothesis that a phenomenon of psychic life can substitute itself for the mutagenic events that must take place in the cell seems to me to be much less probable. However, I belong to the ranks of the practitioners, not the theoreticians, much less the ideologists. If I can be convinced that combining psychotherapy with conventional treatments increases the chances of success ever so little, I will immediately refer my patients to the psychotherapists.

3

❀❀❀

The Cancers of
the Human Species

Experiments can provide us with important information on the causes of cancers in a particular species of animal. Unfortunately, it is risky to extrapolate such information from one species to another. A substance that is carcinogenic in the mouse may be totally harmless in the guinea pig or rabbit. That is why, if we are to discover the causes of cancers in human beings, we must analyze ever more minutely the conditions under which they appear. Such analysis, while still very fragmentary, has given rise to a new and important discipline, the epidemiology of cancer, which studies the distribution of malignant tumors according to the patient's geographical location, ethnic origin, social and occupational status, mode of life, eating habits, intake of toxic substances, and even sexual habits. Thanks to the data collected and analyzed by the epidemiologists, it is now possible to establish increasingly precise correlations between certain external or internal factors and the incidence of various cancers. The existence of such correlations does not always mean that there is a linear relation of cause and effect, but it does throw light on the conditions under which malignant tumors develop. As we shall see, these conditions are many and the skein is not easy to unravel. But there is no doubt that this is a promising avenue of research. A few examples of the epidemiological approach will show how it works, why it is useful, and what difficulties it entails.

The first piece of epidemiological information naturally relates to the incidence of cancers in the total population and the changes in that incidence over time. To the (relatively limited) extent that we can trust statistics in this area, the number of new cases in France is about 160,000 per year, while annual deaths are from 110,000 to 120,000. A comparison of these two figures gives us a very approximate value for the number of cures: around 30 percent. This is less than is generally reported in encouraging public statements. More important, it is less than could be obtained at this time.

In any event, the total incidence of cancer in France and in every country for which we have valid statistics is rising. But it does not automatically follow that cancer is a disease of civilization, although this is true to a certain extent. We must not forget that many diseases that were once fatal can now be cured, and that for that reason alone, the incidence of the others increases, not only relatively but absolutely. How many of us will die of cancer after the age of sixty who a century ago would have died of tuberculosis or rheumatic fever or tetanus before the age of thirty?

Cancers occur much more often in the latter part of life than during the years of youth. Is that, as some believe, because there is a weakening of immunity—in particular, a weakening of the functions of the thymus? Is it because the reproductive program contained in the DNA of the cells "wears out"? Or is it rather that, whatever the causes may be, they must accumulate and work together for many years before a cancer appears? There are some weighty arguments in favor of this last hypothesis. The most important one, which we will come back to later, relates simply to the long duration of latency. There are certain cancers that are known to be caused by chemical agents. They may appear as long as twenty years after the cessation of contact with the dangerous substance. Another argument is based on the form of the curve that expresses incidence as a function of age. Without going into detail, I will simply say that for most cancers, the shape of this curve is compatible with a need for multiple mutations, independent of each other, the probability of which increases with age.

The real incidence of cancer is probably much higher than it appears.

While in a group of 100,000 men of seventy, 200 cancers of the prostate were discovered, systematic studies made during autopsies following death from entirely different causes revealed the presence of undetected microscopic cancers in 15 percent of the subjects. No one knows how many of these cancers would have become evident if the patient had survived longer, but what is certain is that the curves never show a decrease of incidence with age. Their shape implies that if human beings lived to be a hundred and fifty, the frequency of all types of cancer would continue to rise until that age. This can be explained if we assume that the causes work in combination over a period of time. One might regard cancer not as a disease that strikes by accident but as an almost inevitable consequence of aging, and therefore as a disease destined to afflict all those whom advances in hygiene or medicine save from an early death.

I have already used the word "mutation" several times. But should we not consider it a minor miracle that mutations don't occur more often in a world exposed to radiations and chemical influences of every kind? Is it not extraordinary that the program should be transmitted intact from one generation of cells to the next? In fact, if we take into account the vast chain of probabilities, we must stop considering cancer as something abnormal. I here reiterate my conviction that we are dealing with an event that is extremely frequent, habitual, and increasingly probable with the passage of time. In most cases, it is aborted, either because the immunologic police are on the job or because the mutation is too monstrous to survive. But one day it takes root. From this point of view, struggling against cancer means not just fighting an occasional enemy who strikes at random and "unjustly." It means learning little by little to master the very conditions of life, its maintenance and equilibrium at the level of the cell and at the level of the great overall regulatory mechanisms. There is no doubt that the definitive victory over cancer will represent a giant step toward the significant prolongation of individual human life.

Turning to the organs most often affected, we find that the lung, the large intestine, and the female breast are together responsible for half of all cancers—which, incidentally, points the way for our efforts at detection. In males, cancer occurs more often before twenty and after sixty; in females it is more frequent between those two ages, because of the incidence of cancers of the breast and uterus. But these last are curable much more often than are the cancers to which males are particularly subject—lung cancer, for instance; hence the higher mortality among men. Obviously, it's very interesting to study the curve of incidence of the various cancers to see which are increasing and which decreasing in certain geographical areas. In France, for example, it is clear that for the past several years cancers of the stomach have been decreasing, while cancers of the lung have been increasing very rapidly. Does this mean that the causes of the one are diminishing while the causes of the other are on the rise? Or does it mean rather that, within the framework of a relatively fixed number of cancers of all types, the patient who might formerly have developed a stomach cancer at the age of sixty does not have time to do so because at fifty he developed a lung cancer? It is difficult to know.

To give the reader some idea of relative frequencies, here are some figures borrowed from the British, who regularly publish useful statistics. Out of 333 cases for 10,000 men per year, lung cancers represent 29 percent of the total, while out of 300 cases for 100,000 women, breast cancers represent 24 percent. Those are the major causes of cancer morbidity in the human species, and their incidence is mounting. In England and Wales, as in France, we are witnessing a slow decline in cancers of the stomach, but the number of cancers of the esophagus, pancreas, and large intestine is rising. Cancers of the ovaries are increasing by 15 percent every ten years. Two more figures: It is estimated that in 1979 there will be more than 700,000 new cases of cancer in the United States, of which about 90,000 will be breast cancers. Those who want to abandon research, on the totally false pretext that it has accomplished nothing, and to give financial support to prevention instead, should reflect on those figures. There is no known way of preventing breast cancer, whereas we already have treatments for it that are effective and, above all, perfectible.

Tumors of the esophagus are four hundred times more frequent in Rhodesia and Turkmenistan than in Europe and the United States. Cancers of the stomach are observed nearly twenty times more often in Japan and in certain tribes of South Africa than in North America. In Texas, cancers of the skin are a hundred times more frequent in whites than in blacks. Burkitt's lymphoma, which is exceedingly rare in Europe, is frequent in tropical Africa and in New Guinea. Chronic lymphatic leukemia, common in Europe, the United States, and Israel, is very rare in Asia. Fifteen times more cancers of the cervix are recorded in Newcastle than in Liverpool. Lung cancer is much more common in Finland and Scotland than in Sweden and France, and in the United States it occurs more often in blacks than in whites. The existence of such striking differences leads us to think that there are particular causes at work, and those causes are being sought in a great many different factors. It is not an easy undertaking, especially since the geographic survey is far from complete. Besides, it must be broken down not only by country but by region. In the United States there are three to four times more stomach cancers in the Southwest than in the Northeast.

Later I will analyze in detail the role of tobacco and the relationship between maternity and breast cancer. But observation has brought to light an enormous number of other factors that are more or less clearly linked to cancer. A recent study conducted in Nebraska shows that cancer of the esophagus is significantly more frequent among the poor, while cancer of the colon is more frequent among the well-to-do, whose diet is richer in proteins and fats and poorer in cereals. Cancers of the pancreas seem to be more common in urban than in rural populations, which might indicate that research should be done on the possible responsibility of certain pollutants. Cancer of the uterine cervix is observed more often in women whose sexual activity began before the age of eighteen. It is practically nonexistent in communities of nuns and relatively infrequent in Jewish women (the possible role of circumcision of the husband has been discussed).

Melanomas of the skin are most often observed in regions where the sun is very strong, and more often in subjects with light skin. A high consumption of alcohol significantly increases the incidence of cancers of the pharynx, the esophagus, the lung, and the liver, and perhaps also of the pancreas and prostate. The consumption of certain seeds of high oil content, like the peanut, is linked to a particularly high incidence of cancers of the liver. Apparently, this is because of a certain fungus, *Aspergillus flavus,* which is a parasite of the oily seeds and grows best in a tropical climate. The toxins of this fungus have been found to be carcinogenic in the rat.

It would be easy to multiply such examples. The systematic research and increasingly refined analysis of incidence, tumor by tumor, as a function of an infinite number of variables in the environment is a difficult task. But a great number of teams are applying themselves to it, and the information they have gathered has already had considerable impact on the elucidation of the causes of cancers and the development of preventive measures. Yet it would be a mistake to assume that these correlations represent a simple relationship of cause and effect and that congenital factors play no role. There are populations that emigrate, as, for example, Jews of different nationalities who emigrate to Israel, or Japanese who emigrate to the United States. The first generation imports its "incidence profile" without modification. The third generation has almost—but not entirely—the same incidence profile as the population of the adopted country, which sometimes differs widely from the first. In these cases, local habits—eating habits in particular, probably—interact with innate characteristics and finally triumph over them.

When we are dealing with specific chemical agents, it is easier to make progress, because the deductions made on the basis of observations of human pathology can be supplemented by experimentation with animals. But we must still remember that not all species are equally sensitive to chemical carcinogens. The difference seems to depend on whether or not each species has the power to absorb the molecules of the chemical agents and to break them down into harmless fragments, or on the contrary, to split into carcinogenic fragments substances that elsewhere, when they remain whole, have no effect. Nonetheless, it has been possible to indict thousands of substances, both synthetic and natural, complex and simple: arsenic, aluminum, iron, tars, hormones, plastics, dyes, and so forth.

Research is further complicated by the considerable time it often takes for a given substance to cause a cancer to develop. Asbestos is responsible for certain cancers of the pleura. But they appear only after ten to twenty years of exposure. There are thousands of occupations that expose workers to the inhalation of asbestos fibers. Fortunately, only a few workers are affected. However, concentrations of these pleural cancers have been discovered in the residential suburbs downwind from factories in which asbestos is handled.

The first occupational cancer was described in 1775 in England. It was cancer of the scrotum in little chimney sweeps, induced by the tars contained in soot. The workers in certain dye factories are exposed to cancers of the bladder that are caused by beta-naphthylamine. Not a year passes without new chemical substances being at least suspected of inducing cancers. The growing pollution of air and food on the planet is probably partly responsible. Many research teams are studying these forms of pollution. Various food colorings have already been identified and prohibited. Plastic wrappings are being closely scrutinized. Some investigators think that the depolymerization of polyvinyl chloride, under heat and light, produces carcinogenic agents. Even certain medicines may be carcinogenic: many of the drugs successfully used in chemotherapy to treat cancer in human beings induce cancers in some animal species, partly because they have an immunosuppressive effect.

We can get some sense of the difficulty of the problem when we recall that it sometimes takes twenty years for malignant tumors to appear under the influence of a particular agent. But it is clear that, at the very least, it is the duty of the pharmaceutical companies to make sure that none of the drugs they recommend for regular use in the treatment of a chronic disease is carcinogenic in the usual animal species. The cyclamates, noncaloric sweeteners, were taken off the market because they induced cancers in mice. We have no idea what their effect might have been on human beings. But prudence quite rightly prevailed. Here we must give full credit to the U.S. Food and Drug Administration, a fierce and all-powerful watchdog which, acting with complete independence, has the authority to ban drugs, additives, or cosmetics, old or new, after the severest tests, and which doesn't hesitate to do so. Its decisions are sometimes contested, but in this area it is clearly better to err on the side of caution.

There is no point in listing all the carcinogenic agents that have been identified in various animal species, but we welcome the advent of Bruce Ames's test, which makes it possible to evaluate the capacity of any given chemical agent to induce mutations in certain bacteria. The bacteria reproduce every few hours, in appropriate environments, so the mutagenic capacity is readily revealed. This capacity is roughly parallel to the capacity to produce cancers. Not all mutagens necessarily produce cancers in animals. Not all carcinogens necessarily produce mutations in bacteria. Furthermore, not all carcinogens have an effect on human beings. Nevertheless, there is a sufficient correlation for us to consider this test very promising, although we know that the effects of the elimination of a carcinogenic agent will not be felt for some fifteen years, when the number of cancers it causes will be reduced.

Ionizing radiations present the same paradox that we spoke of in connection with anticancer chemotherapies. The radiations, which are so useful under specific conditions for the treatment and cure of cancers, are also undeniably carcinogenic. Since 1902 we have known about the superficial cancers of radiologists and those who handle radiological equipment, and such persons have been advised to be on the alert and to take certain precautions. But since then we have observed cancers, superficial or deep, in patients who have been given radiation for benign lesions in doses that were inappropriate and too strong. We have discovered that cancers of all types appear more frequently in subjects whose mothers received even small doses of abdominal radiation when they were pregnant.

Above all, there has been the terrible human experiment of Hiroshima. Constant cooperation in the field between Japanese and American teams over the past thirty years has made it possible to discover, first, a veritable epidemic of leukemia—an epidemic that began early and lasted a long time—and then, in recent years, an increase in the incidence of cancers of the thyroid among survivors.

Fortunately, it is certain that the natural environmental radioactivity in the world is very far from having reached the threshold amounts that are considered dangerous. But it is equally certain that at a time when we are developing a nuclear technology, mankind should reflect on the possible dangers of moving in this direction. (Although we must also bear in mind that certain hydrocarbons produced by the chemical processing of petroleum are likewise carcinogenic.)

There is still no direct categorical proof that viruses cause cancers in human beings. But it is clearly established that they are responsible for a great many experimental tumors. Viruses are transmitted in two ways: horizontally and vertically. Horizontally, animals contaminate each other, and at least in "domesticated" tumors, cancer is commonly transmitted to healthy animals by the injection of acellular filtrates.

Vertically, viruses are transmitted to descendants, through the mother's milk in the case of certain cancers of mice, or even through the genomes or chromosomal material contained in the germinal cell. Cancers of this latter sort are hereditary in the strict sense of the word.

In examining these facts, we must remember that we are talking not about spontaneous tumors but about tumors that are transmitted in species or strains which have been selected for generations with a view to such transmission, and also that, in most cases, the animals in which they are induced have to be very young.

In spontaneous tumors of human beings, viruses have not yet been found, although indirect evidence—immunological evidence in particular—has been presented. It is possible that the hereditary material, DNA, carries information which, chemically translated, becomes a virus that can be isolated morphologically. Or it may be that an outside carcinogenic virus, made of RNA, can, with the help of an enzyme called reverse transcriptase, inject into the DNA carcinogenic information which, repressed for generations, is one day able to find expression —that is, to produce the cancerous mutation that will perpetuate itself.

Research in this area is being actively pursued, and in 1975 Nobel Prizes were awarded to three specialists working along these lines. The discovery of human viruses that were definitely carcinogenic would mean that there is at least a theoretical possibility of vaccination against cancer—unless hundreds of different viruses are discovered. However, there is no proof that cancers are contagious. If they were, doctors, nurses, and spouses would be affected with a frequency that could not escape attention. If contamination does exist, it must encounter control measures in healthy subjects that prevent cancers from appearing. This is another way of saying what is obvious to epidemiologists: several causes have to be combined.

Cancer is not a hereditary disease—that is, one transmitted from generation to generation according to the usual laws governing the transmission of genetic disorders. The probability that the descendants of a cancer patient will have cancers is slight, but it is not nonexistent. Descendants of subjects who have been afflicted with certain types of cancers are exposed to a higher risk than the rest of the population. It is useful for them to know this, since early detection may contribute to their cure. Among these types of tumors are the retinoblastomas (childhood tumors of the eye, very often curable), certain skin cancers, including a particular variety of malignant melanomas, and breast cancers. Breast cancers appearing in young women before menopause have a family incidence that is definitely higher than that of breast cancers appearing later in life. The difference is small but, as the statisticians say, significant. And if breast cancers are found in the medical history on both sides of the family, the risk is even higher, and the tumor appears earlier in life. This is also true for some intestinal cancers related to a hereditary disease, for a small number of cancers of the uterus, and even for cancers of the lung. Smokers who have had a parent with lung cancer are fourteen times more likely to have lung cancer themselves than smokers whose parents did not have the disease.

In short, although cancer is not automatically transmitted by heredity, there is a greater risk for certain organs if there is a family history of the disease. Furthermore, there are without question families in which tumors of the breast, ovary, intestine, or brain appear from one generation to the next more often than in the rest of the population. And it is not impossible that the accumulation of cases in certain geographical areas with populations of low mobility can be attributed to an extended network of family relations—that is, to consanguinity.

It is hard to say why this is so. The number of children of cancer patients who are themselves stricken with the disease is not nearly high enough to be compatible with hereditary transmission. If cancer were hereditary, we would expect to find tumors in a substantial proportion of descendants. The figure would have to be on the order of 25 percent at the very least. It is actually between 2 and 10 percent, which is already considerable but implies that two or more factors must be combined for the tumor to develop. It is possible that the vulnerability —whatever that word may ultimately mean—is transmitted for a particular tissue and that a virus or chemical agent or other phenomenon must also intervene to make the tumor appear.

In other cases, an immunologic insufficiency is congenital and perhaps hereditary. There are certain rare families in which several generations are successively stricken with cancers that appear in unrelated organs but are all associated with an immunologic deficiency. These families are valuable subjects of study for those who are trying to elucidate the genetic aspects of cancer.

Lastly, it is well known that diseases involving chromosomic malformations caused by mutations or accidents are accompanied by cancers more often than pure chance would dictate. This is the case, for example, with mongolism, where the risk of associated leukemia is very high. The exact nature of the connections between cancer and genetics is yet to be determined. But studies in this area may pave the way for early detection, and perhaps for prevention through genetic counseling.

Everything I have said so far shows that several factors must be combined to create a cancer, or conditions favorable to a cancer; that is what makes the problem so complex. Let us see what is known about these combinations of causal factors as they relate to the two commonest types of tumors: breast cancers and lung cancers.

Breast cancers

It has long been known that mammary cancer in mice is caused by Bittner's virus, which is transmitted through milk. In the milk of certain women, viral particles have been found that closely resemble this animal virus, and such particles are found much more frequently when there is a family history of breast cancer. Furthermore, in the blood of certain women there is an antibody that neutralizes Bittner's virus.

Unfortunately, the decrease in breast feeding over the past several decades has not been followed by a decrease in the incidence of breast cancer. This shows that other factors must be involved, or else—as is possible—that the virus is incorporated in the DNA. That would mean that in certain cases, the genetic information responsible for cancer is transmitted as soon as fertilization takes place and doesn't express itself until much later, in an appropriate context and under the influence of an appropriate stimulus. Many researchers are working on this hypothesis.

The role of the hormone folliculin in triggering breast cancer in mice was demonstrated several decades ago, and certain researchers tend to attribute human breast cancers to an imbalance between folliculin and progesterone. We know for a fact that the history of a woman's endocrine glands and reproductive organs has a distinct influence on the incidence of breast cancer. It occurs more often in women whose menopause comes late, who have not given birth or nursed (nuns, for example), or who reached puberty early. It has, however, been impossible so far to identify a specific hormonal profile typical of breast-cancer patients. (I should mention in passing that no evidence has yet been found to indicate that hormonal contraceptives are in any way responsible for cancer.) Lastly, "receptors" for folliculin have been discovered in the cells of certain breast cancers. These cancers seem to be more sensitive to the various anti-estrogenic therapies than those in which such receptors are absent.

This brief discussion of viral and hormonal factors shows how complex the matter is. It is possible that there are two different types of breast cancer, one caused by a virus and the other by a hormonal imbalance—and both are subject to possible hereditary influences. But it is also possible that the expression of a carcinogenic virus is affected by hormonal influences. It is up to the epidemiologists and experimenters to answer these questions in the years to come. The answers might have consequences for both treatment and detection, and even for prevention.

Lung cancers

In lung cancers the role of carcinogenic factors is better established. Tobacco is the great purveyor of cancers of the lung, and its role has been demonstrated beyond a doubt, both by experimentation with animals and by epidemiological studies in man. The tars contained in the products of combustion of tobacco induce skin cancers when they are simply painted on the skin of animals. They produce lung cancers in animals that are made to smoke or merely to live in a smoky atmosphere—which, by the way, points up the risk incurred by nonsmokers who live in an environment where other persons smoke. As for human beings, here are some facts: in a group of British doctors who agreed twenty years ago to be the subjects of a long-range study, mortality from lung cancer decreased by 30 percent among those who gave up using tobacco, while it increased by 25 percent among those who continued to smoke. It has even been proved that the risk for a smoker begins to decrease five years after he or she has given up the habit, and that after ten years of abstention it becomes the same as for a nonsmoker—that is, negligible.

A famous survey done in Los Angeles compared the general population with the Seventh-Day Adventists, who neither drink nor smoke. Over several years, the latter presented the same number of cancers of the prostate, the colon, the breast, and the uterus as was predicted by the statisticians on the basis of the epidemiological data collected on the rest of the inhabitants. However, instead of the eleven lung cancers that were expected, only one was recorded. The risk of lung cancer for a nonsmoker is not zero, but it is thirty times less than the risk for a man who for fifteen or twenty years has been smoking two packs of cigarettes a day.

It is true that we are beginning to identify other carcinogens, such as asbestos, chrome, the emanations from uranium mines (occupational cancer), and other more recent pollutants. But even though all these risks are cumulative, it is still better to be a nonsmoker in Paris than to smoke forty cigarettes a day in the mountain pastures of Lozère. The positions taken recently by officials of the tobacco industry in France are in absolute contradiction to the entire body of scientific facts.

But exposure to tobacco is not the only factor. I have already said that a smoker who had a parent who had lung cancer is fourteen times more likely than another smoker to develop a cancer himself. A very important recent discovery accounts for both the chemical-carcinogen theory of bronchial cancer and the genetic theory, and also explains why there are smokers without lung cancer and lung cancers without smoke. This is the discovery of the enzyme aryl-hydrocarbon hydroxylase, which has the property of "activating" tobacco tars by purifying, as it were, the dangerous part of the molecule, which thus gains easier access to the target cells. It has been demonstrated that the distribution of this enzyme is governed by simple genetic laws. Those persons who have none are much less likely to develop cancer than those who have it in large quantities. Let us hope that a routine test will soon be devised that will enable us to identify an especially high-risk group of smokers. What each member of the group does with that information will then be up to the individual.

In connection with possible genetic factors, we should also mention the veritable epidemic of lung cancer among American blacks who smoke, an epidemic whose causes are unknown.

The influence of sex also can't be denied. The increase in lung cancer in women and in men has been parallel over the past thirty years, but all things, and especially the amount of smoking, being equal, the rates among women are much lower. Could this be due to hormonal differences? Or to Y chromosomes, which determine masculinity and might carry greater vulnerability? These are important questions which epidemiological surveys might be able to answer. Let us also point out that researchers in Marseilles have discovered that a genetically determined blood protein is unevenly distributed between lung-cancer patients and other subjects.

The existence of a viral factor has never been definitely established, but in this connection we should recall certain curious geographical differences: for example, the extremely high incidence of lung cancer in northern Europe (Finland, Scotland) and in New Zealand. Some epidemiologists have made a connection between the path traced by points of unusually high incidence of bronchial cancer and the migratory route of certain birds well known to be carriers of pathogenic viruses and even of various carcinogens.

Lastly, I want to note another disturbing phenomenon: it seems that a British researcher has discovered a group of subjects with a high risk of lung cancer, a group composed of persons who are now between sixty and sixty-nine, which is basically responsible for the overall increase in incidence. As the members of this group grow older, they take the risk with them, along with the problems it poses, because the older a patient is, the less susceptible he is to radical surgery. The rate of lung cancer among younger subjects apparently remains relatively stable. If this tendency is confirmed, what does it mean? What mysterious event took place thirty years ago whose effect was added to the risk of smoking in men who were then thirty to forty?

It is clear even from the brief discussions in this chapter that we can't expect a prompt and unequivocal answer to the question of what causes cancer. Unfortunately, the statements that appear in the press every ten years, announcing that an isolated, misunderstood genius has discovered the cancer microbe, are inspired by either charlatanism or paranoia. We must expect that, for each type of cancer, the epidemiologists will gradually identify a multiplicity of risk factors, which will then be more or less confirmed by experimental models. That in itself will be an immense boon to humanity, because it will enable us to define certain high-risk groups and to concentrate our efforts at detection and prevention on the persons who stand in the greatest danger. So far as prevention is concerned, however, I hope I may be permitted to express my pessimism.

The pollution that accompanies industrial development, which we have not yet learned to master, arouses vehement indignation in some people. But for all that, people do not stop administering carcinogens to themselves—tobacco and alcohol, for example. Indeed, the demand for them is growing. Similarly, those who deplore the consumer society do not practice frugality—if they did, it would have the additional virtue of being an ideal remedy for the increase in arteriosclerosis.

It seems that, instead, people have decided to go on poisoning themselves while they wait for doctors to find the magic pill that will enable them to do so without risk. This attitude reflects a touching confidence in science that is diametrically opposed to the views of the advocates of zero growth. I share this confidence, at least from a certain point of view. Otherwise, I would not have written this book. Furthermore, I believe we will never return to the simple ways of earlier times. The automobile will not be replaced by the bicycle, but it will become electric. Meat will continue to be preserved, but with noncarcinogenic additives. Cancer will be curable. Wisdom will not spread throughout the land. We will be able to satisfy people's needs, but never their desires.

4

❁❁❁

The Natural History
of Cancers

It is not enough to be able to describe a tumor—that is, to distinguish it from healthy tissue. If we want to have an effect on it, we must understand the dynamics of what goes on inside it, the laws that govern its history, the different stages of its development. How does a cancer grow? How fast? Are there periods of latency or regression?

These are very important questions. However, for a variety of reasons of an epistemological nature, the scientific community began asking them only recently—a quarter of a century ago, at most. Doctors approached cancer primarily as pathologists, looking at it from the static point of view of morphology, and most specialists are still content to do so. Yet it is obvious today that knowledge of the natural history of cancers is an absolute prerequisite for the therapist who wants to change the development of a tumor. The study of these aspects of the disease is far from complete, but it has already revealed important facts, which the reader should know in order to understand the following chapters dealing with the various kinds of treatment. Here again, while awaiting the decisive discoveries of the scientists, doctors have set about taking advantage of their own clinical and experimental observations. We shall see that they have not fared too badly.

The life of an "active" cancer cell is from one to ten days between the time it is born and the time it divides into two daughter cells. If we assume an average life of five days, this means that the tumor's volume should double every five days, an absolutely explosive rate of growth. We do observe growth of this order in acute childhood leukemia, which accounts for the rapid evolution of that disease in the absence of treatment. But in the usual cancers of the breast, the lung, the colon, and the various other organs, it is very different. Cancers in human beings are slow diseases which last several years. I should like to explain how we came to accept this notion as a fact, and what its various consequences are.

Certain tumors lend themselves particularly well to a study of their rate of growth. These are the spherical tumors which develop in the lungs and can be measured on X-ray photographs to the millimeter. This does not mean, of course, that we measure them to see how they evolve without treating them. But we have several means available for evaluating their rate of growth. The first is simply to compare their diameter at the time they are discovered with their diameter on the photograph taken just before the operation. There is a certain lapse of time between the two because of the various examinations that have to be made. This, however, provides only two measurements, relatively close together, on the basis of which one can make only a crude estimate. But in certain cases, patients refuse to be treated. That happened during a study made in Philadelphia in which, over a period of years, a large population of adult male smokers were given chest X-rays for early detection. Those subjects who were discovered to have cancer were informed of the diagnosis, and it was suggested that they undergo surgery. Some of them refused any kind of treatment but agreed to have photographs taken at regular intervals, which made it possible to measure the tumor and establish a growth curve. In other cases, where there were many bilateral tumors, it was impossible to attempt surgery or radiotherapy. Before there were medical treatments for cancer, patients in this category were merely given drugs that made them more comfortable but had no effect on the growth of the tumors; these could therefore be measured by successive X-rays over a more or less extended period of time. I have looked up such files in the archives of several hospitals and analyzed them to discover the rates of growth for various types of cancers and to determine whether or not there are laws that govern those rates.

The time that it takes for a tumor to double in volume varies between the extremes of ten and four hundred days, with an average of about ninety days. If it takes three months for a roughly spherical tumor to double in volume, that means that its diameter doubles in nine months, which is frequently the case for a whole series of cancers.

The fact that it was possible to draw up curves of spontaneous growth for thousands of tumors enabled researchers to discover a phenomenon that at first was very surprising: during the period when tumors in human beings are visible and can be observed clinically, their doubling time is approximately constant; there is a geometric progression. Volume v at time t_1 becomes $2v$ at t_2, $4v$ at t_3, $8v$ at t_4, etc. This constancy was first demonstrated twenty years ago by an American team. Many doctors still find it startling and are disturbed by the idea that a cancer's growth is not an anarchic, unpredictable phenomenon. I must confess that I personally am not bothered by the fact that any natural phenomenon can be described by an equation. It is the contrary that seems to me to be exceedingly rare and suspicious. In any event, I can't resist the temptation of recounting how we were put on the track of these studies.

In May 1968, I was an associate professor working at Laënnec Hospital in Paris as assistant to Roger Even. The student uprising was raging, and it aroused mixed emotions in me. It was at the height of the agitation that a series of references led me to an article by Collins that had appeared in an American journal in 1956 and then passed into oblivion. On the basis of a series of observations, it established the constancy of the doubling time of pulmonary tumors. I was immediately fascinated by the possibility of bringing order into a phenomenon that until then had seemed chaotic. Furthermore, I glimpsed the possibility of predicting, on the basis of a given point in the evolution of the disease, what would happen if it was not treated—that is, of comparing the results of treatment to the situation that would have developed in the absence of treatment. But I had to make sure that Collins's theory was based on fact, as is not always the case. I confided my thoughts to my resident, Philippe Chahinian, who had done advanced studies in mathematics and had the necessary turn of mind for this sort of investigation.

We had at the time a patient with a measurable tumor, the metastasis of a cancer of the rectum, who had just been sent to us accompanied by several successive X-rays that enabled us to establish the rate of growth. Chahinian took the file home with him and the next morning came back discouraged. "If the doubling time were constant," he said, "there should already have been a small but visible pulmonary metastasis when he had the operation on the rectum three years ago. But in that case, they wouldn't have operated on him. Therefore Collins was mistaken."

Undismayed, I tried to get hold of the chest X-ray the surgeons had surely made at the time of the operation. It was in a hospital in the suburbs. The postal workers were on strike, so I sent a student for it —he agreed to tear himself away from the revolution for one day. When he got back, Chahinian and I had a bit of excitement. The tumor was indeed there and of the predicted size—eight millimeters in diameter—but it was behind a rib, where it had escaped attention. So Collins's theory was becoming plausible. We spent a good part of those famous days of May examining data, making calculations, and writing equations for the growth of tumors, which we were later to publish. Since that time, we have devoted much effort to this area and have developed a tool that is taking its place in the evaluation of different therapeutic strategies.

Corrections have been supplied, in particular by experimenters who, without calling into question the fundamental fact that growth is a regular phenomenon, have formulated a law, or mathematical expression, that is slightly different from ours and very interesting. Indeed, it is now definitely established that from the time of injection of a single cancer cell until the death of the animal, the rate of growth decreases according to a regular law. A tumor that takes two days to double in volume when it has a diameter of one millimeter takes ten days to double in volume when it has reached a diameter of one centimeter, two weeks when its diameter has reached two centimeters, and so forth. In other words, the rate of development decreases with time, and it decreases according to a predictable pattern, which can be described by a mathematical function.

How are we to reconcile this fact with what clinicians observe—that is, a doubling time that is constant? The answer is that the observable period in human beings, under the conditions described above, is only a small part of the total evolution of a tumor. During this period, the doubling time can be considered as constant, give or take errors in measurement. Nevertheless, we can't deduce the tumor's "date of birth" simply by extrapolating the curve to the beginning, since we know that in the past its growth was more rapid than it is now.

To approach the very important problem of a tumor's "lifetime," we must first ask how many times it has doubled before being discovered. There is an approximate answer to this. If, for ease of calculation, we assume that the average diameter of a cancer cell is ten-thousandths of a millimeter—an assumption perfectly compatible with reality—it follows that in order to reach a diameter of one centimeter, the tumor will have had to double in volume thirty times. Therefore we say that a tumor one centimeter in diameter has reached its thirtieth doubling. It so happens that this thirtieth doubling is a very important point in the history of a tumor, because this is the earliest stage at which tumors of the deep organs can be detected. Teams of doctors and radiologists have patiently verified this fact. At that point there are approximately one billion cells in the tumor. Clinical observations show that it is very rare for an untreated tumor to go beyond the fortieth doubling—that is, to reach a diameter of ten centimeters, corresponding to 1,000 billion cells. Usually, fatal complications have arisen before then. Thus deep tumors, which are often difficult to detect and which produce symptoms relatively late, are discovered at the earliest at the thirtieth doubling, and the fatal conclusion is reached before the fortieth. That means that for these tumors, we are at present able to offer treatment only in the last quarter of the evolution of the disease, which is terribly late.

To estimate the date when a given tumor started, we may take the example of a doubling time of one hundred days, calculated for a tumor one centimeter in diameter. If the rate of growth was constant, it would place the birth of the tumor eight years earlier, but we know that that is too long. Calculation shows that the tumor began between six and four years before it was discovered.

The doubling time of one hundred days is rather long for cancers of the lung (whose average is sixty days), but it is frequent in cancers of the breast, kidney, prostate, and so forth, which shows how much time we could gain if we had another indicator besides the symptoms, which generally appear too late. To underline the advantages of gaining time, I need only point out the following: by taking systematic Pap smears of the uterine cervix—an extremely simple, painless procedure that consists of collecting exfoliated cells on a glass slide—gynecologists are able to detect tumors that are still invisible, less than one millimeter in diameter—that is, having doubled less than twenty times. And surgery alone is sufficient to cure 90 percent of such tumors. To be sure, the cervix happens to be an organ that lends itself particularly well to this kind of cytological detection; that is, it is possible to study isolated cells rather than the fragments of organized tissue that are necessary for biopsies.

It is an extraordinarily complex problem to detect deep cancers before the thirtieth doubling, and one that is far from being solved. It might be possible to make a systematic effort to detect the disease at least in members of high-risk groups, either by regularly checking the blood or organ secretions for biological substances that would reveal the presence of a tumor at its inception (such substances are beginning to be found), or by regularly examining cells found in bodily secretions or collected by the smear procedure, as in the Pap test. One detection campaign of this sort, well known to specialists, has, however, served only to increase their perplexity.

Miners of uranium who also smoke run a very high risk of developing lung cancer. As smokers, they spit in the morning. Trained cytologists who examine their expectorations can identify suspicious cells. If they find such cells in several successive examinations, they can be almost certain. Yet X-rays and bronchoscopies are normal, because the tumor has not yet reached the visible stage. What is to be done? It is possible to tell from samples taken under bronchoscopy from which lung and even from which lobe the cancer cells come. But what then? Some cautious specialists have advised waiting. Years later, a cancer has appeared that has proved fatal. Others, more daring, have operated. Naturally, no cancer could be detected by microscopic examination of the tissue excised. Was it necessary to operate and make the subject run even a minimal risk? Other miners who were not operated on have not developed cancer after a number of years. This may be because of cytological errors (the technique has built-in causes of error) or—who knows?—it may be because the tumors in question were very new and the organism was able to combat and finally destroy them.

We can see from this example that highly refined detection is almost impossible, and that in any event it poses further problems that are beyond our present resources. If we had drugs that were both effective and safe, they could be administered to high-risk persons such as the miners described. But chemotherapy and immunotherapy should not yet be used—and, so far as I know, they never have been—to treat potential cases: the risk of a treatment should be proportionate to the risk of what might happen in the absence of treatment, and subjects cannot be treated at random. But we already have some simple methods of early detection, and it is important to take advantage of them to gain time. Gynecologists, gastroenterologists, specialists in diseases of the lungs, the larynx, the urinary organs, and so forth should examine the target organs in adults every six months or every year, and women themselves should examine their breasts regularly at the end of each menstrual cycle.

In France this "clinical" examination, backed up by simple laboratory tests, is performed in the Social Security centers, not only for insured persons who are invited to come in for check-ups but for anyone who wants to come. And, of course, such examinations should be done by all general practitioners. If they are not done often enough, it is usually the patient's fault. The man who goes to see his doctor for rheumatism would be surprised to have his prostate examined. This attitude must change, and adults must ask their doctors for annual check-ups. I want to emphasize that it is not so much biological tests that are wanted but manual examination and possibly X-rays. These would at least make it possible to detect at the thirtieth doubling tumors that otherwise would not reveal their presence until the thirty-fourth or thirty-fifth.

What goes on inside a growing tumor? The rate of growth measured is only a crude phenomenon. If we want to be able to interfere with the tumor's development, to slow it down, arrest it, or better yet, destroy it, we must try to find out more about what takes place inside it.

First of all, there is a discrepancy to be explained: the discrepancy between a doubling time of three months, for example, and a generation time (that is, the time between the birth of a cell and its division) of three days. If all the cells divided, and if they all remained in the tumor, the doubling time and the generation time would be identical, and all cancers would be galloping diseases. Fortunately, this is by no means the case. Why?

In order to find an answer to this question, a whole scientific discipline has evolved, with its own means of investigation and calculation. This is the discipline of cell kinetics, which experimental oncologists, if they have not invented it from scratch, have at least greatly expanded. There is no need to go into details here. Suffice it to say that a tumor loses cells, and that not all of those that remain proliferate. Cells are lost in two ways: first, some are so greatly undernourished in comparison with their neighbors that they die without having multiplied; second, many are sloughed off into the bloodstream. (I will return later to this second phenomenon, which is absolutely decisive for the prognosis of the disease.)

The reason that some tumor cells fail to proliferate seems to be that certain cells, which receive a relatively poor supply of nutritive material, survive but do not divide. In principle, proliferating cells pass through the following cycle: a phase called G_1, during which biochemical phenomena that we do not completely understand occur; then an S phase of synthesis of DNA, during which the quantity of DNA doubles; then another G phase, G_2, preparatory to division; and finally a division phase, M (for mitosis). Cells that are not proliferating are said to be in phase G_0 or a very prolonged G_1. Various experiments have shown that the proportion of nonproliferating cells may be as high as 95 percent of the total at any given time. When I add that the chief medical and radiation therapies can be effective only on cells that are proliferating, the reader will understand how important this figure is and how useful it would be to have ways of making resting cells "enter the cycle." Researchers are aware of this problem, but it has not yet been solved. We already know however, as will be seen later, that certain drugs are more active on one phase of the cycle than another. And this fact is of great significance in establishing chemotherapeutic strategies.

Another point should be emphasized here. The growth of a tumor appears to be a compromise between the generation time, the coefficient of proliferation or growth fraction, and the percentage of cell losses. The tumor increases in volume by the multiplication of the proliferating cells. It diminishes because of the losses, while the non-proliferating fraction tends to maintain a stable volume. This compromise must be governed by a law, since the doubling time is subject to a regular variation and therefore has a determined value. It follows that for a given doubling time, measured in a particular case, the above parameters cannot vary independently of each other. Along with other teams, I and my colleagues have studied this problem. Michel Duchatellier, a talented young mathematician with a doctorate in physics (who worked on a volunteer basis, because it was impossible to find a line on the budget for him at Lariboisière, until he finally became discouraged and went into industry), showed us the relation between these factors and how we could exploit it in treatment.

The cell losses can be very high. Not all the cells manufactured by the tumor serve its growth. If the coefficient of proliferation is high, the losses can be as much as 95 percent of each new generation: the tumor amputates itself. One reason is that not all the cells manage to attach themselves to the fibrin coagulum that supports the tumor and contributes to its organization. Couldn't we give a little push and nudge that figure up from 95 to 100 percent—that is, stop all growth? Naturally, this idea has occurred to many investigators, especially those who are concerned with the relations between cancer cells and the system of blood coagulation. Certain experiments, but not all, have shown that safe anticoagulants could significantly slow the growth of tumors. More than ten years ago, an English doctor noted that cancers occur less frequently and grow more slowly in patients who are taking anticoagulants for prolonged periods for heart diseases. And of course aspirin comes to mind, because it blocks one of the mechanisms of coagulation. Aspirin, however, also suppresses the activity of the lymphocytes. Nothing is simple. But the researchers are imaginative, and they don't give up easily . . .

A cancer is serious to the extent that it spreads to other parts of the body. If tumors remained localized, we would have only to remove them to have a 100 percent record of cures. Everyone knows that this is not possible. In more than 80 percent of cases, it is the distant metastases that kill, not the original tumor. Where do metastases come from? Obviously, from the cells that the tumor sloughs off into the bloodstream. Most of them die there. Others die in the organs where they stop, very probably because of an immunologic attack by the macrophages, as has recently been demonstrated for the lung. But some find the necessary conditions for survival and development.

It is evident that the risk of metastases depends on the length of time that has elapsed and the number of cells that have been placed in circulation. This number can be increased by inopportune manipulation of the tumor, repeated examinations, and so forth. But it depends chiefly on the tumor's rate of growth. That has been confirmed experimentally. Tumors that grow rapidly give rise to many and early metastases. Those that grow slowly produce fewer and later ones.

When we know that a tumor has existed for years and been sloughing off cells all that time, it's a safe bet that it has produced metastases. And where metastases are concerned, we must be guided by the probabilities; we must not feel that our responsibility ends with excision of the visible tumor but must remember that everything possible should be done to hold in check or destroy the invisible tumor, the more serious one, which is represented by all the metastases that are still microscopic. Their rate of growth is related to that of the primary tumor, but it also depends on the tissue in which the metastases develop, the pressure of the surrounding tissue, the amount of blood that reaches them, and many other factors. Consequently, we're unable to predict these growth rates at present.

We can't measure all tumors—far from it. How, then, are we to evaluate their rate of growth, which is so important for the therapist? Personally, I haven't found any connection between a tumor's rate of growth and the way it looks under the microscope. But an American statistician has made a simple observation: the visit to the doctor that results in the discovery of the tumor is precipitated earlier by symptoms connected with rapid growth than it is by symptoms connected with slow growth. If this is true, and if it is also true that slow growth means a better long-range prognosis than rapid growth, we should find that patients who are operated on when their symptoms have lasted for more than six months recover more often than those whose symptoms are of recent origin. Paradoxical as it seems, this statement is amply confirmed by statistics relating to several hundred cases of various tumors. It is therefore possible, if not to measure, at least to make a rough estimate of the rate of evolution of most malignant tumors when they are discovered.

I have learned a great deal over the past ten years from living at a crossroads of disciplines. It's true that my ambiguous position at Lariboisière creates administrative problems that are sometimes depressing (and sometimes amusing). But there are also advantages to the "different" point of view that, particularly as a lung specialist, I bring to my work with cancer.

Through its respiratory function, the lung filters all the pollutants that enter the organism through the air. But not all of them stop in the bronchi, as witness cancers of the bladder that are caused by tobacco. Some undergo either beneficial or harmful chemical transformations in the lung. The study of the purifying mechanisms of the deep lung—a study to which members of the French school, and notably Jacques Chrétien and Cyr Voisin, are contributing so much—is becoming an important division of epidemiology and carcinogenesis, and it may one day become the point of departure for a real means of prevention.

Through its circulatory function, the lung receives and filters the vast majority of cancer cells that have been liberated from the tumor and are looking for a home. Some simple calculations we've made show that it destroys a great number of them, sometimes even all. Sometimes, too, the lung is vanquished in the end and allows itself to be invaded. In certain cases, it resists invasion in all but a few sites. The studies we're conducting with a view to reinforcing the power of the lungs to purify out cancer cells that have come from other organs (and not just external pollutants) may eventually have implications for oncology in general.

Similarly, thanks to the fact that pulmonary metastases are, as I've said, particularly easy to measure, my special vantage point has enabled me to study the spontaneous growth of tumors and the possibilities of predicting their response to various treatments. Lastly, an investigation we're conducting at Lariboisière is beginning to show that tobacco—which depresses tissue immunity—does not merely cause primary lung cancers. It seems that by lowering the lung's power to purify tumor cells, it is also responsible for a great number of metastases in other cancers of adulthood.

I have based this chapter on my personal experience in interdisciplinary medicine. In my opinion, interdisciplinary work does not mean the meeting of specialists in different disciplines, but rather the meeting of different disciplines in the same individual—an adventure that our system discourages, when it does not absolutely forbid it.

5

✿✿✿

Prevention and Detection

Once again, I should stress that this book does not attempt to survey all the problems raised by cancer, but rather to emphasize the short-comings of cancer treatment today. Nevertheless, I want to say a few words about prevention and detection here.

It is possible that someday there will be a general vaccination campaign to prevent certain cancers, but I'll take the risk of saying that I don't think it probable. The epidemiology of tumors in human beings has little connection with the transmissibility of tumors induced by viruses in specially bred laboratory animals.

At present, there are two ways to prevent cancer. The first is to try —with the help of the Ames test, for example—to eliminate mutagenic agents from everything that can be ingested or breathed in. No effort should be spared to accomplish this. We will never know how successful we have been, because the cancers that would have been induced by those agents won't appear, but we can easily resign ourselves to remaining in ignorance. It is important to remember, however, that the Ames test does not detect 100 percent of carcinogenic agents; also, it may reveal that some common natural substances are harmful. "Nature" is not always benevolent: arsenic in its natural state is carcinogenic, and so are asbestos and uranium.

The second method of prevention, and the more rational one, would consist of eliminating substances we already know to be carcinogenic, such as tobacco, and to a lesser degree, alcohol. It is perfectly obvious that we won't be able to do this. The obstacles aren't just economic. These poisons provide pleasure and feed deep-seated fantasies, and their ill effects do not afflict all consumers to the same degree. There's something appealingly naïve in the belief that through education we will one day be able to persuade people to abandon them entirely. If humanity were collectively responsive to the counsel of wisdom, we would probably have noticed some sign of it by now. Therefore, while we should encourage prevention campaigns, I don't think we should depend upon them to solve the problem of cancer in the next few generations.

Still, let me make one more appeal against tobacco. The reader will remember what I said at the end of the previous chapter. In my opinion, it is probable that in addition to its direct carcinogenic role as a generator of primary lung cancers, tobacco promotes the pulmonary diffusion of other cancers by paralyzing the local means of immunologic defense. I think that smoking is as dangerous for a woman who has a high likelihood of breast cancer as for a man with chronic bronchitis. I therefore applaud without reservation the courageous campaign of our Minister of Public Health. We must not expect immediate or complete results. But it will be a great day when tobacco advertising is banned, and when personalities who have prestige in the eyes of young people are no longer allowed to appear on television or in films with a cigarette in their hand. As a physician, I am necessarily an advocate of the possible, and not a seeker after absolutes. Every adolescent who is persuaded to refuse tobacco will represent a victory, as well as a saving for society. (I am grateful I have no political responsibilities and don't have to worry about the economic fate of the workers in the tobacco industry.)

More attention should be paid to detection, although it is not a panacea either. As we have seen, the goal is to identify cancers before they have metastasized but when they are already visible and thus can be removed. This is possible, but only for a few organs—the cervix is one of the rare examples. That there is a direct correlation between a tumor's size and its seriousness has been amply confirmed, but there are many exceptions to the rule, particularly in the case of small cancers with a rapid growth rate. For reasons that will be immediately evident to readers of a statistical turn of mind, a random detection program will reveal more slow tumors than rapid ones, which means more curable tumors than dangerous ones (a paradox I shall not pursue). Nevertheless, whatever the gravity of a tumor, it is always advisable to treat it as early as possible. Opinions vary from one country to another as to the "profitability" of cancer-detection campaigns, and I will refrain from trying to settle the question. But there can be no argument that, at the very least, information should be widely disseminated, so that each individual can not only recognize symptoms from the start, but also know if—because of heredity, occupation, or addiction—he or she belongs to a high-risk group. As a description of high-risk groups emerges, it should, of course, be taught first of all to physicians. Since there is no regular instruction in oncology in our medical schools, that will not be easy. In the meantime, it seems to me that cooperation between the high-risk subject and his doctor is a good—and immediately available—way of ensuring early detection of a great number of cancers.

I want to conclude this chapter, and the first part of the book, by stressing the fact that, for the reasons I have already given, no effort at prevention or detection will either eradicate cancer or make it curable. There will continue to be innumerable cases, many of which will be impossible to detect early. Furthermore, while early detection may make treatment more successful, it doesn't enable us to obtain acceptable percentages of cure—far from it. There is therefore an enormous need for research to discover better methods of treating tumors. Indeed, this is clearly the problem on which we should concentrate our efforts. It would be an incomprehensible mistake to turn away from therapeutic research on the ground that the progress we are making is too slow.

Part Two

❀❀❀

CONVENTIONAL METHODS OF TREATMENT

For more than a century we have been removing cancers surgically; for three-quarters of a century we have been irradiating them. These techniques have saved a great many patients, and they will save more. So there is no question of being opposed to them or of wanting to limit the kinds of cases in which they are used. Quite the contrary. I want here to examine the results obtained by these techniques in order to show why they are useful. I also want to show how they can complement, and be complemented by, modern medical treatments. Some surgeons and radiologists unnecessarily restrict their specialties to a limited number of clinical situations. For my part, I hope that when surgery and radiation are brought into contact with the new medical oncology, their range of application will rapidly expand.

6

❀❀❀

Surgery

Surgery was the first weapon to be used against cancer, and in the vast majority of cases it continues, alas, to be the only one. A patient with a tumor that appears localized and so placed that it can be excised without risking the patient's life is operated upon. This practice, which came into being at a time when we knew nothing about the natural history of cancers, consists of removing the visible tumor and leaving the invisible one. Either the surgeon wagers that in this particular case there is no secondary tumor and he has intervened in time, or he trusts to nature to control the micrometastases, which are the great danger for the future. Or he may take a palliative approach from the beginning, on the theory that removing the primary, visible tumor will prolong the patient's life and save him needless suffering, and that nothing more can be done. In addition, since the patient is not usually informed of the diagnosis, successful surgery can give him the illusion of cure.

But it must be understood that surgery is, and will continue to be, an extremely valuable weapon against cancer. Except, perhaps, in the case of certain cancers highly responsive to radiation, every cancer patient who can be operated on should be. There is no alternative, for we don't yet have a magic pill that enables us to sterilize a tumor. It's absolutely untrue that surgical removal of a tumor provokes an explosion of hidden metastases. There are some cancers that are growing so rapidly that they must be "cooled" by radiation before they are removed. There are others—certain "small cell" bronchial cancers, for example—that surgeons systematically refuse to operate on because they know that metastases will appear within three months anyway. But these cases are rare. Usually, surgery is necessary, and it is tragic that operable patients are sometimes advised against it. In the last few years surgical techniques have made impressive progress in every area, and even advanced age is no longer an insuperable obstacle. I think it absurd to "compare" the results of surgery with the results of other procedures and to consider various techniques competitive, when they are in fact complementary. Nevertheless, if one were to restrict oneself to a single weapon, as most doctors do, one would have to choose surgery.

I've already discussed the meaning of "cure" in connection with cancer. The word is used arbitrarily and improperly by surgeons, and it's better to talk about lengths of survival than about percentages of cure—bearing in mind, of course, that to obtain prolonged postoperative survival is to render an immense service to the patient even if, in the strictly scientific sense, he hasn't been cured.

The figures on length of survival vary somewhat from one team to another, and of course depend on the selection of cases—that is, on the daring and determination of the surgeons. A cautious team that operates only on small lung cancers which have no involvement of mediastinal lymph nodes will achieve more brilliant results than a team with a different philosophy. But the results will apply to a smaller percentage of total cases.

We must also remember that figures provided by surgeons apply only to cases in which they actually removed the tumor, not to the cases in which they merely tried to do so. The rate of operability also varies according to the team and the local conditions encountered by a surgeon during an operation. Furthermore, statistics on postoperative survival don't include patients who died within thirty days after the operation. The full significance of this becomes apparent when we recall that, because of the frequent invasion of contiguous tissues and involvement of lymph nodes and blood vessels, cancer surgery entails much more serious complications than surgery of the same organs for nonmalignant disorders.

Lastly, the retrospective surveys that surgeons make in order to establish curves for survival include cases that have been lost track of and others in which, while it is known that the patient is still alive, it can't be determined whether or not he's free from metastases or recurrence of the original tumor. The few figures given in the table, which are averages based on statistics from many different countries, will give the reader a general idea of the results obtained by surgery.

Type of tumor	Five-year survival (in %)	Ten-year survival (in %)
Cancer of the breast without involvement of the lymph nodes	80	50
Cancer of the breast with involvement of the lymph nodes	50	25
Cancer of the stomach	25	10
Cancer of the lung	25	10
Cancer of the kidney	30	5
Cancer of the uterine cervix { Stage I	85	
Stage II	60	
Stage III	35	
Stage IV	10	

We have seen that these results relate to groups that are generally highly selected. For example, as I've indicated, only about 15 percent of lung cancers are operable at the time they are diagnosed. These figures are therefore an accurate measure of the place of surgery alone in the arsenal of anticancer weapons. Surgery has innumerable successes to its credit, if we use the rates of five-year survival as our criterion. At the same time, it has very serious limitations, since the high rates occur in cases where the tumor is discovered early and is still relatively small. These, we must remember, are cases of "external" cancers, those affecting organs accessible to regular smears, like the cervix, or to palpation, like the breast. The deep cancers, which are much more difficult to detect, give poorer results, both in terms of the rate of operability and in terms of postoperative survival.

I should also point out that the table indicates the size of certain tumors but not their rate of growth. The rate of growth is a difficult factor to evaluate, and surgeons aren't yet in the habit of taking it into account. Our team has studied this factor at length, and our data—which support the findings of American teams—indicate that there is a direct correlation between the rate of growth before the operation and the speed with which metastases appear. The faster a tumor is developing, the less surgery affects the course of the disease. Surgeons are sometimes puzzled by cases of lightning evolution after the removal of a very small tumor, as they also are, on occasion, by cases of long survival after the excision of a very voluminous one. But such cases only confirm the fact that if we want to refine our prognosis, and hence our therapeutic strategy, we must take into account not only the size of the tumor but also its rate of growth.

One of our studies shows very clearly that surgery alone does not radically alter the natural history of cancers. Unfortunately, the shape of the curves for postoperative survival in a large population of patients is dependent upon the statistical distribution of doubling times in that same population. The patients who are "cured" are those in whom the doubling time of the tumor is very long, and who therefore take a long time to rebuild a population of threatening cancer cells. Removing the visible portion of the tumor is a very effective act in that it brings the disease back to an earlier point in time. If we remove ten billion cells and leave behind only one million, we bring the cancer back from the thirty-third doubling to the twentieth, and the slower the disease was, the more time we gain by so doing. But we have by no means eliminated the tumor. Thirteen doublings later, it will have reached the same point as before the operation.

The powerlessness of surgery to cure cancer is further illustrated, moreover, by a striking fact. Twenty percent at most of patients who die after having had surgery succumb to an isolated local recurrence, while 80 percent die of distant metastases, which existed in germ, of course, before the operation. Thus if we were able to perfect local treatment, we might achieve an additional 20 percent of successes, but that would still leave 80 percent of failures. When in 1969 I set forth these facts, based on many statistics, in a French medical journal, I received a request from an American medical journal for permission to reproduce the article in its entirety; at the same time, I received indignant letters from French surgeons. I suppose their indignation is no less lively today. Do they pretend to believe that I was condemning surgery when I urged only—and explicitly—that surgery be complemented by general treatments? There are also some who think these complementary treatments are more harmful than the disease itself, without having had the slightest personal experience of them, or—what is worse—after having applied such treatments themselves when they were not competent to do so. Others have no definite opinion on the subject but can't bear to have anyone raise questions about practices they have always followed.

There is another advantage to surgery. Along with many other teams, we have observed that in a third of the cases where a tumor is removed, there is a marked improvement in the patient's immunological status. A very long study has shown us that these same patients have a better long-range prognosis than the others. It's clear from this that surgery is not only a means of removing a dangerous mass of tumor cells from the organism, but also a means of manipulating the immunological condition so that it has a favorable influence on the course of the disease. This is what Georges Mathé and his students mean when they say that "the surgeon practices immunotherapy without knowing he is doing so."

I am so far from being opposed to cancer surgery that I want to sum up a few proposals designed to improve its results. These suggestions aren't new. They are, however, generally followed haphazardly, whereas they should be carefully studied and applied in accordance with an overall strategy.

1. No cancer surgery should be undertaken until a specialist in medical oncology has seen the patient, subjected him to various examinations, assigned him to one of the prognostic subgroups, and elabo-

rated a strategy in which surgery plays an important part, but not the only one and not necessarily the first in order of time. If the patient is to receive postoperative treatment, he should learn of it before the operation so that it doesn't come as a surprise. And the doctor should make sure that it's possible for the patient to obtain the treatment in his particular geographical location.

2. Whenever possible, given the organ in question, the surgeons should reexamine the problem of first tying off the blood vessels. This procedure is designed to prevent the trauma of surgery from putting in circulation millions of malignant cells, some of which may in the long run produce metastases. Surgeons often speak of surgery that is "carcinologically satisfactory"—in other words, complete—but their concern that it should be so does not necessarily lead them to take this often simple precaution. It is up to them, if they wish, to evaluate its impact on experimental models.

3. The question of administering anticoagulants—or agents that inhibit platelet aggregation—during the postoperative period and over the long term is acquiring increasingly great theoretical importance. Cancer patients have a tendency to hypercoagulation, and circulating cancer cells form metastases more easily in areas of hypercoagulation. Isolated but consistent studies by American surgical teams have repeatedly shown that the postoperative prognosis for cancer patients is markedly better when heparin, a powerful anticoagulant, is prescribed. It is true that after a difficult operation anticoagulants can be dangerous. It is also true, however, that certain techniques for inhibiting platelet aggregation or the accumulation of fibrin could be used instead. But how long will we have to wait to find out for certain how useful these treatments are? I've always been dumbfounded by situations in which a team proclaims an important result that no one else verifies. Thus for years a potential advance may not be brought into general practice, or a useless or even harmful procedure may continue to be occasionally applied. One solution might be to establish a central body whose responsibility it would be to propose contracts for studies that would clear up unanswered questions, and to solicit bids from teams interested in undertaking them.

4. If surgery in certain deep locations is to be followed by radiation, radio-opaque clips should be placed around the site of the excision or

around any portion of the tumor it has been impossible to remove. This procedure can be of first importance, because it will greatly increase the radiotherapist's precision. In the United States, I've seen surgeons spend two hours thus circumscribing lesions that couldn't be removed. Many French hospitals, both public and private, lack the necessary equipment, although it is by no means expensive, simply because the surgeons have never requested it.

5. The surgeon's report of the operation must give a minute description of the lesion. The radiotherapist, the chemotherapist, and the internist, who will see the patient later, can't do without it, nor can the statisticians. But many a report that expatiates at length upon the difficulties encountered and the surgeon's emotions says not a word about the number of lymph nodes examined and their exact location and arrangement. There is an international classification for tumors, called the T.N.M. (tumor, lymph nodes, metastasis), that makes it possible to give each cancer a fairly precise classification on the basis of which, in part, a prognosis can be made and a course of treatment determined. In France, cancer surgeons are familiar with this classification and use it. General surgeons, whether in private practice or attached to hospitals, regularly ignore it, so their reports of cancer operations are unintelligible and useless. All these attitudes stem from the semi-conscious belief that where the knight of the scalpel has passed, the tumor is slain—or if it comes back to life, only God can intervene, not mortal men. Clearly, in view of the increasing incidence of cancers, all surgeons should be given a minimum of training in the matter, and soon.

The points discussed above place stricter demands on the surgeon, but they do not conflict with his deep-seated convictions or the concept that has been instilled in him of "carcinologically satisfactory" surgery —a notion that comes straight from the nineteenth century. However, there is more to be said about surgery and surgeons in the light of current ideas about the natural history of tumors.

In the United States I have seen abdominal surgery performed which was so extensive that it was not so much a therapeutic act as an acrobatic feat on the part of the surgeon and such that I personally would prefer not to survive rather than to survive in such a condition.

From this point of view, the common sense of the French surgeons seems to me to be far preferable to the pioneering attitude of certain specialized American surgeons, even if—and I must emphasize this— the patients, who are always forewarned, consent to these procedures. On the other hand, certain operations so extensive that many surgeons would think them preposterous are followed by very satisfactory results. Abbey Smith, a British thoracic surgeon, and Olivier Monod in France, for example, have an impressive record of results from such operations. We must remember, in this connection, that the prognosis depends in part on the rate of growth. The laborious excision of a large tumor and the neighboring organs it has invaded may be worthwhile if the cancer's evolution has been slow.

When oncologists speak of "reductive surgery," they mean partial operations designed to reduce the size of a tumor. These don't make much sense unless they are followed by further treatment, but in that case they can be very helpful. The smaller the tumor, the more effective chemotherapy is. That is why a physician may ask a surgeon to reduce the size of a tumor that can't be completely removed before he begins medical treatment. My surgeon friends—strange as it may seem, I have many!—are not easily persuaded to perform such operations. Of course, if they are consulted first, they're even less likely to mention the possibility of performing reductive surgery and then referring the patient to a medical oncologist. In this regard, too, they will have to change.

The problem of limited surgery comes up particularly in connection with breast cancer, and I shall return to the subject in detail when discussing combined strategies. But I should also like to say a word about it here. More than a hundred years ago, William S. Halsted developed an operation for radical mastectomy, including removal of the breast, the two underlying pectoral muscles, and all the lymph nodes in the armpit, at the cost of extensive skin loss and considerable mutilation. This operation reflected the conditions of a time when radical surgery was an absolute necessity—there was no radiotherapy —and when surgeons were consulted much later than they are today and had to deal with more voluminous tumors that had always spread to the lymph nodes and were sometimes ulcerated. It is truly remarkable that in spite of increasingly early diagnosis and the almost universal application of postoperative radiotherapy, a majority of surgeons throughout the world persist in performing an operation that is so mutilating. There has been protest against the practice, and certain surgeons perform more limited operations. Here again, the opposing camps inveigh against each other instead of agreeing upon trials that would make it possible to reach a definitive conclusion.

So far as I know, only one reliable trial has been conducted in this area, by my friend Bernard Fisher in the United States, and its conclusion was that the results of Halsted's operation and of a similar one that respected the pectoral muscles were identical. Is it possible to go further? Perhaps, but only if we take great precautions that will be discussed in the chapter on clinical trials. It is high time we got together to obtain answers to these questions, because if—as I personally suspect —more limited surgery is equally effective, there's no justification for pursuing a policy that causes women so much suffering.

Let me say a few words about the question of systematic lymph node resection, in order to show how complex the problem is and how subject to change our present notions about treatment are. A breast cancer sends cells into the lymph nodes of the armpit. The lymph nodes are therefore systematically removed. If they are "negative," the postoperative prognosis is better than if they are positive, and everyone leaves it at that. Yet we know that it is in the lymph nodes that the macrophages and the lymphocytes receive and exploit the antigenic information that will lead to specific immunity. Would it not be better to leave the lymph nodes intact? Would it not be better even to respect those that are microscopically invaded and remove only the ones where metastases are obvious? No one yet knows, but the question has been raised, following certain experimental observations, such as those of Fisher on breast cancer in rats, and certain clinical observations, such as those of my friend Pierre Banzet in Paris regarding melanomas of the limbs. When will we have a clear and conclusive answer to this important question?

A patient has so large a tumor that it is judged inoperable, and he is given palliative treatment. The treatment is particularly successful. The tumor diminishes in size. Why not remove it then and continue treatment?

One of my young patients was operated on in 1963 for a primary tumor of the testicle. Two months later he had a second operation, for a pulmonary metastasis, performed by a friend of mine who is a particularly determined thoracic surgeon. But three months after the second operation another pulmonary metastasis appeared, and the discouraged surgeon turned the patient over to me for chemotherapy to slow its advance. After six months of treatment the growth of the metastasis had been arrested, and no new one had appeared. I had all the trouble in the world to persuade the surgeon to operate a third time. Finally he did so. We continued chemotherapy for three years. This patient is now cured and has started a family.

It's also possible to introduce surgery into a therapeutic program in which it couldn't be included at first. Physicians who specialize in cancer do this all the time. But when will surgeons, who are consulted first in the vast majority of cases, instead of declaring the patient inoperable and sending him back to his family doctor with a sigh, automatically refer him to a chemotherapist and ask to see him again after a few weeks or months to reevaluate the possibility of surgery?

When I speak of repeated surgery, it is surgery on metastases that I have in mind, as in the example above. Certain surgeons practice it; it should be done more often. At Memorial Hospital for Cancer and Allied Diseases in New York City, I saw a young man from whom surgeons had removed twenty-seven pulmonary metastases of an osteosarcoma (in two stages). The surgeons' obstinacy had triumphed over the disease. Two years later no new metastasis had appeared. This may be an extreme example, but it is certain that the surgeon who specializes in cancer, who is educated as to the other therapeutic possibilities and trained in an offensive approach, can obtain much better results than the general surgeon who is technically perfect but intellectually ill prepared for the battle against cancer.

In 1955, Vangensteen, an American surgeon, proposed that patients who had been successfully operated on for cancer of the stomach or intestine should be reoperated on every six months or every year for "inspection," so that any regional recurrences that had appeared in the interim could be removed. His proposal caused much merriment on this side of the Atlantic. But Vangensteen reported results which showed that from 20 to 30 percent of the patients were "saved" by this procedure. It is true that American patients are generally told their diagnosis and know what is at stake. It is also true that cancers do not usually remain regional. But in future such a practice might come to seem less extraordinary than it does to certain persons today.

Let me conclude by saying that surgery, an important weapon if ever there was one, is far from having made its last contribution to the treatment of cancer. Technical progress in this area depends on advances in surgical technique as a whole. But long-range progress depends on surgeons' training in cancer, on their imagination, and on their spirit of cooperation. In addition, surgeons must turn toward integrated strategies. This may take away some of their prestige, but it will enable them to serve many more patients than they do today. Not long ago the various specialists concerned still regarded the different anticancer weapons as competitive. It will have taken twenty years for some—still too few—to begin to think of them as complementary. How long will it take before all patients have the benefit of the best possible treatment as soon as they consult a doctor?

It has been said that truth never triumphs, but that the champions of error finally die. I can't believe that it will always be so in medicine. The speed with which we are advancing demands the greatest flexibility of mind and the ability to renounce preconceived opinions in favor of more objective views. One of the tasks of those who are planning various reforms in the selection of doctors should be to detect the individuals who correspond to that profile. I've always told my students that I was in favor of a pitiless selection of medical students—that is, that I was for eliminating the narrow-minded, the unstable, the careless, the ideologists, the lovers of intellectual comfort.

But this sort of selection would accomplish nothing if it wasn't accompanied by precise, modern instruction. So far as cancer surgery is concerned, there's a crying need for such instruction. And it's obvious that a part of it should be dispensed not by the surgeons themselves but by those of us who request their services, the internists or medical oncologists, and also by kineticists, histologists, immunologists, and statisticians. Then and only then will we see an immediate increase in the effectiveness of surgery in the treatment of cancer. Once again, technical perfection isn't at issue. Our surgeons are equal to those in any country in the world on the most difficult cases. But they are living on theories that were current fifteen to twenty years ago, and there have been many advances in medicine since then.

7

❀❀❀

Radiation

Chronologically, radiation was the second weapon to be used against cancer. X-rays, discovered in 1895 by Wilhelm Roentgen, were applied the next year by Despeignes, in Lyons, to an inoperable cancer of the stomach. Since then, there has been an uninterrupted succession of scientific and technical discoveries down to the present time, when gamma rays produced in accelerators are used, and most recently, equipment has been developed to deliver high-speed neutrons and pi mesons. In addition, radiotherapists use radioactive bodies, which they implant in the tumor itself, and radioisotopes, which are introduced into the organism and seek out their target—the skeleton, for example, or the thyroid gland. With all these techniques at its disposal, radiotherapy is a very valuable weapon that can be expected to have an expanding role in the future, thanks to better cooperation between radiologists and other specialists.

The particles delivered in radiotherapy transfer their energy to electrons which ionize the matter they reach—that is, which produce free or ionized chemical radicals. For example, they ionize water, which constitutes about 80 percent of the organic environment, by separating it into the radicals H, OH, and so forth. Of course they also ionize the "solid" constituents of cytoplasm, RNA and DNA. This ionization damages the molecules, weakens them, and leads to recombinations with the oxygen available in the environment. Thus changes occur in the biological properties of the molecules. Some of these changes cause the cell to die, others make it impossible for it to divide, and still others lead to extinction at a future time, the descendants of the affected cell dying out after three or four generations. We know many biochemical and genetic details of these injuries, and already they have shown us how complex the phenomenon is. A cell does not die because it bursts apart, or because its proteins suddenly coagulate, but because of a series of delicate events that take place over a period of time and are combated by certain mechanisms of self-repair.

Radiotherapy in its modern form is now the treatment of choice in the early stages of Hodgkin's disease (five-year survival: 80 percent). It is very effective in seminomas of the testicles, and in cancer of the cervix and the prostate. In cases of small breast tumors, it gives results that many investigators consider comparable to those of surgery. A certain number of cancers of the nasopharynx have also proved very sensitive to radiotherapy. I am talking about treatment that aims to cure—that is, the treatment of cases that are seen early and are operable in principle, but for which ionizing radiation is used instead of surgery, as a definitive local-regional treatment. In cases of this sort, radiotherapy sometimes gives brilliant results. Yet, apart from Hodgkin's disease and lymphosarcoma, there is much disagreement as to its effectiveness—indeed, there have been no conclusive trials—and many physicians prefer surgery, despite the mutilation it entails, because it has the advantage of making a clean sweep: total sterilization by radiation often remains problematical.

As a palliative treatment, radiotherapy is absolutely irreplaceable for localized but inoperable tumors, such as certain tumors of the lung, esophagus, pancreas, colon, breast, and so forth. In such cases the aim is not to bring about a cure, for the tumor is too large, but to obtain at the very least a considerable attenuation of symptoms, often a partial regression of the tumor and the pain it causes, and on occasion even a regression that is apparently complete. In this connection, it is regrettable that radiotherapists don't report their results—as chemotherapists do—in such a way as to differentiate between the percentage of complete regressions and the percentage of objective partial regressions, and to indicate the distribution of length of those regressions. In any event, the results are often only palliative. Radiotherapy suffers from the same limitation as surgery in that it does not affect metastases, and from another limitation as well, which we will analyze later in detail: the difficulty of achieving local sterilization.

The purpose of applying radiotherapy both before and after an operation—a practice that has long been in use—is to perfect the results of surgical excision. This practice is an admission that surgery alone, even when it is visually satisfactory, does not remove everything, and that by combining two different local treatments, we increase the chances of sterilization. If this reasoning is correct, we should observe a reduction in the rate of local recurrences when radiation is added, and no change in the rate of distant metastases, since there is no reason why those should be influenced by an improvement in local treatment.

In fact, we observe something rather different. Local recurrences do diminish in cases of advanced tumors, where there is great danger that malignant cells will have migrated to the lymph nodes of the region or to adjoining tissues. But they do not diminish in cases in which local recurrences are already very rare: a small breast tumor, a peripheral lung tumor. As for distant metastases, certain recent studies have thrown the medical community into confusion by showing that metastases may be more frequent in cases that have received radiation, a finding that could be explained by a pernicious effect of ionizing radiation on immunity. There are still only a few of these studies, and those that do exist are contradictory and highly controversial. But they show that in medicine, logic and deduction cannot take the place of long, honest, empirical studies undertaken with an open mind.

Radiation can cause more or less extensive burns of the skin and mucous membranes; these generally repair themselves in a few weeks, and can usually be avoided by experienced radiotherapists. Vascular lesions that may appear later are more severe and can cause necrosis and fibrosis with loss of function of the irradiated tissues. The different organs vary in their vulnerability to this sort of complication. The liver, kidneys, and lungs are particularly fragile; the muscles are also susceptible. Even very moderate amounts of radiation of the testicles and ovaries may cause sterilization or induce genetic mutations that will reveal themselves in later generations. It is known that radiation has a teratogenic effect: if it is applied before the third month of fetal life, there is a slight but not negligible risk of malformation. The practice of giving regular X-rays to women who are three months pregnant has been abandoned. (It was required by Social Security at a time when the risk of not recognizing tuberculosis in the mother was much higher and more serious than the risk—which no one suspected anyway—of damaging the child or its later offspring.)

Lastly, radiation is carcinogenic at smaller doses than those which immediately injure tissues. The radiologists were the first to suffer from this complication. A few years ago it was learned that irradiation of the thyroid region during childhood is dangerous and, in a not inconsiderable number of cases, induces cancers in the adult.

It may seem curious to use ionizing radiation to treat diseases that can also be caused precisely by ionizing radiation. But the paradox is more apparent than real. Weak doses of radiation are mutagenic and can start the chain of phenomena that, over a period of several years, leads to cancer. Strong doses are destructive, and more so to tissues that are proliferating rapidly than to healthy neighboring tissues, and it is logical to exploit this property. Nevertheless, one might express concern that the radiation that sterilizes the cancer may induce carcinogenic mutations in the healthy tissue through which it passes. There may be some basis for this concern, and it is up to the radiotherapists to evaluate it precisely, for the benefit of us all. But the risk remains absolutely minute. And if we can sterilize a tumor by radiation today, we must do so, even at the risk of inducing a tumor the day after tomorrow. Sufficient unto the day is the evil thereof.

When a wide area is exposed to radiation, it is impossible to avoid irradiating large portions of the skeleton and hence of the bone marrow in which the different blood-cell lines are formed. The serious bone-marrow deficiency that would result if the entire body was irradiated in sufficient doses is an insurmountable obstacle to such therapy, unless a bone-marrow graft is performed afterward, which is still an exceptional procedure. As I have already mentioned, it has recently appeared that radiation can also cause a severe and prolonged immune deficiency. This is true for radiation of the thymus, the organ in which the T-lymphocytes are processed, and hence for radiation of certain tumors of the lung, esophagus, and breast, among others. But it is also true of the radiation of large abdominal areas, which affects an extensive system of lymph nodes, bones, and blood vessels. The more the patient's immunological status deteriorates, the greater becomes the risk of both regional and distant dissemination. From this point of view, we are beginning to suspect that radiotherapy is a two-edged sword, and that it would be well to think about possible ways of countering this very serious disadvantage.

Fortunately, healthy tissues and tumors have a different sensitivity to rays. Certain tissues—intestinal mucous membranes, for example—proliferate faster than tumors and can therefore regenerate themselves more quickly, between two successive sessions of radiotherapy. Others proliferate only as needed to repair losses, and are therefore much less vulnerable to radiation than the tumors, which do not have this feedback mechanism of repair, but on the contrary, proliferate constantly. It is nonetheless true that it is impossible to irradiate a tumor without damaging the surrounding healthy tissues. It is the responsibility of the radiotherapist, with the help of calculations and complicated machines, to establish the best compromise between effectiveness and tolerance. But it is still only a compromise. One would have to sacrifice too much healthy tissue, tissue that is often indispensable, in order to be sure of sterilizing the tumor. It can't always be done.

Certain phenomena combine to limit the effect of ionizing radiation on tumors. When an area is bombarded with rays, the destructive events they produce are not equally divided among all the cells. Some cells undergo two, three, or four events when one would have sufficed. Thirty-seven percent are not affected at all. The next time, 37 percent of this 37 percent are spared. And so on. Consequently, the radiotherapist wears himself out trying to hit the last cells and can't do so unless he totally destroys the neighboring tissues. If one cell out of ten thousand escapes, and if the tumor had 10^{11} cells (that is, weighed 100 grams) in the beginning, there remain 10^7 cells, which continue to proliferate and will become 10^{11} cells again in thirteen doublings. The probability of radically sterilizing a tumor by radiotherapy rises in direct proportion with the risks one takes with regard to the healthy tissues, but it is never equal to 1.

The cell in phase S, the phase when it is synthesizing DNA, is much more resistant to radiation than the cell in phase M. Unfortunately, for statistical reasons, there are ten to twenty times more cells in phase S than in phase M at any given time. Cells in phases G_1 and G_2 are of an intermediate sensitivity. Cells in a very prolonged G_1 phase are not totally insensitive to radiation, therefore, and that gives us a precious opportunity to reduce the number of nonproliferating cells. Still, even if all the other conditions for effectiveness are met, the succession of the various phases of the cycle of division represents an important limitation to radiotherapy.

The presence of oxygen is almost indispensable to the success of radiotherapy, for the oxygenation of the free radicals converts them into compounds that are definitely unsuitable for their intended biological use. But the diffusion of oxygen through the capillaries ceases to be adequate beyond a range of 0.2 millimeters. Certain tumors of insufficient vascularity have areas that are hypo-oxygenated and hence resistant to radiation. That is a great problem for the radiotherapists. We shall see how they try to solve it.

The way in which DNA repairs itself when damaged is a fascinating phenomenon. In both normal cells and tumor cells there are enzymes that recognize in the DNA chain the parts that have undergone chemical damage and cut them out, while other enzymes "sew up" the two fragments, end to end, maintaining the proper order. The repair is sometimes imperfect, and the cell's progeny will suffer. Sometimes it is excellent, and the cell behaves as if nothing had happened. This is a very effective mechanism of radioresistance, although it varies from one tumor to another, from one tissue to another, and perhaps genetically from one individual to another. Certain tumors of the skin, tongue, lips, and so on respond slowly to radiation but are permanently cured. Others—certain sarcomas, for example—melt like snow under the rays of the sun but recur more or less quickly. We can't explain these differences.

Since I am neither a radiobiologist nor a radiotherapist, my notion of the prospects for radiotherapy is no doubt imperfect, and the specialists may not all agree with me. Nevertheless, as a medical oncologist—that is, as a person who needs their services for his patients and who reads many papers in their field—I am interested to see that radiotherapy is not, as some might think, a fixed discipline, but rather one that is making rapid strides and from which we may expect much.

It is important to concentrate the rays on the tumor and to protect healthy tissues, and several methods have been devised to accomplish this. One of them, which has been in use for a long time, consists of employing a cross fire of rays from several directions, in such a way that each intervening portion of healthy tissue penetrated from the skin down receives fewer rays than the tumor itself. Today radiologists using this empirical approach can call upon all the resources of dosimetry. Computers now make it possible to draw the isodose curves, to simulate a clinical situation with an irregular tumor and its particular localization, and to know precisely how the rays will be distributed in and around the tumor. This appears to be a major advance, of such importance that radiotherapy installations that don't have these facilities will soon be outmoded. Another approach would consist of utilizing beams of fast neutrons or pi mesons generated in accelerators; these are more penetrating and can be more selectively localized. Most of the preliminary studies have already been undertaken. We don't know exactly how this heavy artillery—heavy in every sense of the word—will fit into the total arsenal of radiotherapy, but it appears that it will have an important place. Still another procedure is to implant radioactive materials in accessible tumors. Recent innovations here consist of using iridium-192 and cesium-137 instead of radium. As always, there are controversies among specialists. There are probably important advances to be made in the precise localization of the effects of radiation. A Parisian team has acquired a world-wide reputation in this field.

How can we combat radioresistance? It would be ideal if we could inhibit the ligases, the enzymes that repair damaged DNA. We will probably find a way to do that one day by biochemical procedures: certain studies suggest that drugs as simple as caffeine might have the desired effect.

Taking another approach to the problem, investigators have already done a great deal of work on the "oxygen effect." Tests have been conducted of irradiation during and following massive oxygenation of the patient with a mask, under a tent, and even inside a chamber where the pressure can rise to three atmospheres. The tests were not conclusive. But it does not seem that we can use these techniques to surmount the obstacle of oxygen deficiency in the tissues caused by lack of vascularity.

However, other procedures can be summoned to our aid. Various substances, such as synthetic vitamin K, metronidazole, and so forth, concentrate by choice in hypoxic cells and perform the function of oxygen by attaching themselves to free radicals. It will not be easy to measure exactly the increase in effectiveness thus obtained. However, many radiotherapists are devoting themselves to the task, and with all the more enthusiasm because these substances are not harmful. The field of radiosensitizers is wide open.

The difference in sensitivity of the different phases of the cycle is an obstacle that might be overcome if we could find a way to "synchronize" the cells. If we take as the total duration of the cycle twenty-four hours, an S phase of eight hours and an M phase of a half-hour, at any given moment we have one-third of the cells in phase S, or resistant, and one-fiftieth of the cells in phase M, or highly sensitive. We know that in some doses, certain chemical agents that can be utilized in chemotherapy are capable not only of killing cells but also of temporarily arresting others in a given phase. That is the case, for example, with the antimetabolites and the fluoridated pyrimidines, which block cells in phase S. While these substances are active, all the cells reaching phase S from phases G_2, M, and G_1 remain in phase S. When the effect of the chemicals wears off, the cells resume the cycle at the same time and will reach phase M at the same time. They will have been "synchronized." If the radiation treatment is applied at the right time, it will find many more cells in phase M than before synchronization, and its effectiveness will be increased accordingly. Actually, these theoretical propositions are very hard to check. We must extrapolate from results obtained in small animals with small tumors, in which all the parameters are different from those that exist in man. Nevertheless, the idea is certainly one to be pursued. It has already been partly confirmed by clinical studies showing that the synchronization obtained, while it is far from 100 percent, is by no means negligible.

The purpose of splitting the total dose into fractions is not only to combat radioresistance. It is also to increase the difference in effect on

healthy tissues and on tumors. If the patient is to receive a total of
6,000 rads, why break it down into fractions of 200 rads, delivered in
five-minute sessions, five times a week for six weeks? I am almost certain
that it is not merely to keep their weekends free that radiologists treat
their patients only five days a week. But the fact is that the ideal
schedule is not yet known. We know that the larger the fraction that
is administered at one time, the greater the destructive effect, but this
is true for normal tissue as well as for the tumor. We also know that
the shorter the interval between two fractions, the poorer the repair,
but again this is true for both normal and pathological tissues. Continuous irradiation is dangerous to healthy tissues unless we use the technique of implanting the radioactive material in the tumor itself. In
order to optimize the breakdown schedule, we would have to know the
relative kinetics of healthy tissue and tumor tissue in each case, which
is usually impossible. It would be a step forward if radiologists would
take into account the rate of growth of the tumors they irradiate,
instead of calmly applying the same schedule for a tumor with a doubling time of ten days and for one with a doubling time of four hundred
days. It is possible that certain tumors should be irradiated two or three
times in the same day and others only twice a week.

The basic objective is not to improve radiotherapy but to improve
total results. One way to do that is to improve the use of radiotherapy
within an overall strategy employing all the weapons available. Is it
useful to supplement palliative radiotherapy with a course of chemotherapy? Is it possible to use immunoprotection and immunostimula-
tion—before, during, or after radiotherapy—to reduce its immunosuppressive effects without diminishing its antitumor effects? Should we
systematically irradiate areas in which postoperative metastases are
likely to appear, before they do so?

Radiation remains a local treatment, unsuited for the management
of a diffuse disease such as cancer usually is. But this local weapon is
of great value because it can be used where surgery is no longer feasible,
and it can be used against several different metastases where it would
be unwise or impossible to remove them all surgically. It doesn't provide the degree of sterilization that can be achieved with surgery, but
current research is making it increasingly effective. It isn't the weapon

itself that's open to criticism, but some of those who use it, who consider medical treatments as nonexistent or as lesser forms of therapy having only a supporting role in relation to radiation.

A few of the radiologists to whom I refer patients before subjecting them to medical treatment, instead of sending them back to me, tell them that such treatment is unnecessary. Most radiologists do send patients back and are curious to know the results we obtain afterward. But there are not many who spontaneously suggest chemotherapy to a patient whose radiation treatment is coming to an end, even when the risk of recurrence remains very high, as in the case of an inoperable lung cancer, and even when they know that while they may have achieved local control, they have done nothing to protect the patient from metastases at a distance. The opportunities for radiotherapists and medical oncologists to work together are still rare, at least outside of anticancer centers, and the level of communication between them suffers as a result. I hope that new structures can soon be established that will make it easier to exchange information, to adopt a common language, and to eliminate mutual mistrust. The patients have everything to gain from such cooperation.

Recently the radiotherapy journals have contained an increasing number of articles on tests of irradiation of the entire body. Some very encouraging results have been published. These results have been achieved by using weak doses that don't endanger the organism and that allow repopulation of the bone marrow by cells that form the various elements of the blood.

8

❁❁❁❁

Hormone Therapy

Hormone therapy is the first known treatment for cancer that can be administered generally, to the entire organism. It is only slightly toxic, compared to chemotherapy, and it is very tempting intellectually because it offers a means of modifying the internal environment and preventing the growth of cancers that are hormone-dependent. It is therefore interesting to examine the role of sex hormones in cancers of the genital area, in which "antagonistic" hormone therapy can be administered.

No one has been able to present convincing evidence that female hormones have an effect on cancers of the testicle or male hormones on cancers of the ovary. This lack of effect is surprising on the face of it, and it would be worth further study to find the explanation. In any event, it is a fact. However, cancers of the corpus uteri and certain ovarian tumors seem to be improved by progesterone, the second of the female hormones.

Controlling cancer of the prostate is the triumph of hormone therapy. In 1941, Charles B. Huggins showed that castration or the administration of female hormones of the folliculin type could cause cancer of the prostate and its metastases to regress in a very large number of cases. This situation is no doubt a model of what medical treatment of cancer will be in the future, a treatment capable of preventing the growth of a given type of cell without interfering with other cells in the organism. We might wonder, incidentally, how it is that even large and numerous metastases regress in these cases, because while estrogens inhibit the growth of cells that need male hormones to proliferate, they have no destructive effect in and of themselves. It is probable that the immunologic system takes over to finish the job. The fact that estrogens stimulate the macrophages may have something to do with this phenomenon. But the limitations of estrogen therapy in cancer of the prostate and the obstacles it encounters are also interesting to consider. They show the complexity of the problems we confront.

There are cancers of the prostate that are resistant to hormones from the outset. Not all cell lines are equally dependent on the same biochemical environment. Some are completely untouched by the treatment. This sort of uneven reaction to therapy is a common occurrence in oncology, and one that is particularly frustrating.

The fact that certain cancers are affected by female hormones does not mean that they are cured. In the end—fortunately after a very long period of time in some cases—the vast majority fail to respond. Is it because the dependence on hormones gradually disappears? Or is it because hormone-dependent cell lines are destroyed, leaving only those that are resistant? It is possible that both mechanisms are at work.

Not all the effects of estrogens are beneficial. They induce cardiovascular accidents—infarctions, embolisms, apoplexies—because they produce a tendency to hypercoagulation. A recent American study, which appears to be irreproachable, has caused much consternation by showing that patients who were given estrogens derived no benefit whatever from their anticancer properties because of an increased mortality from cardiovascular accidents. No one has yet undertaken the study that would attempt to compensate for this effect by using anticoagulants.

It has long been known that breast cancer can be hormone-dependent. It was proved a few years ago. In certain cases—but not all—cancer cells have receptors for female hormones which make them dependent on those hormones. If the sources of estrogens are eliminated and/or male hormones are administered, the cancers temporarily regress. In these cases, important results can be obtained by removing the sources of estrogens (not only the ovaries but the adrenal glands as well). Surgical excision of the adrenals, however, creates relatively complex problems in maintaining balance in the internal environment. The removal or destruction of the pituitary can also be useful, because it eliminates the pituitary hormones under whose influence estrogens are secreted, and also another hormone as well: prolactin, which seems to accelerate the growth of breast cancers, at least in some cases. But again, this procedure is rarely employed, because of the problems of hormonal balance it creates. That is why, especially after removal of the ovaries, doctors have long preferred to prescribe the male hormone, which is supposed to counteract the effects of the residual estrogens secreted by the adrenals. This procedure is simpler and quite often effective. But it causes a very disagreeable virilization in exchange for a benefit that is usually of short duration. Certain products called "anti-estrogens," which have no virilizing effect whatever, are now being studied. Their configuration deceives the estrogen receptors, which confuse them with estrogens, but they have no hormonal action. We shall soon be able to tell what their place will be in the treatment of breast cancers. The first results are extremely encouraging. For the past year we have been using them at Lariboisière with a success that, I must say, I did not expect. Among our results, which were recently published together with those of a group in Canada and another in Philadelphia, there are some that are simply fascinating: complete and lasting regressions of disseminated lesions.

Very old women can also develop breast cancers. It is generally agreed that more than five years after menopause the quantity of estrogens secreted is absolutely negligible and that these cases are not estrogen-dependent. It has even been suggested that they should be treated by female hormones. And these do sometimes bring about a partial and temporary regression of lesions. Is this because of a direct hormonal effect, immune stimulation, or the blocking of harmful pituitary secretions? Several teams are currently trying to solve this problem. But it should be pointed out that in any event, here as in cancer of the prostate, cases can be "controlled" only for a time, and seldom completely. Even in those breast cancers that are most authentically hormone-dependent, there are undifferentiated cell lines that aren't affected by hormonal changes and that proliferate in spite of endocrine treatments. For these reasons, no matter how brilliant its results may be at times, hormone therapy is not, and will not be, the solution to cancer. But we don't have so many solutions at the moment that we can afford to reject this one. The problem is, rather, how to use hormone therapy in combination with others, especially since it is not very toxic. If we use anti-estrogens to treat a breast cancer in which 10 percent of the cells are hormone-dependent, we won't perceive any result, for it will be masked by the proliferation of the other cell lines. But if we institute treatments that are active on the other lines, that 10 percent may make the difference between success and failure.

There are other endocrine cancers besides cancers of the genitals—for example, those that affect the adrenal glands, the thyroid, or the internal secretion cells of the pancreas. In addition to present methods of combating them, a better understanding of biochemistry may in the future make it possible for us to intervene directly in the hormonal process. Can hormones also have an effect on nonendocrine cancers? We have reason to believe that they can. I have never personally observed the regression of metastases from cancers of the kidney under the influence of progesterone, but many favorable reports have been published, and the question remains on the agenda.

In the distribution or evolution of certain cancers, there are differences between the sexes that are so striking as to suggest that the administration of "antagonistic" hormones might have an effect. Here again, many experimental studies are in progress, and the question is one to be pursued.

Lastly, certain hormones have nonspecific effects. The male hormone, for example, seems to protect bone marrow or to stimulate the repair of damage to bone marrow caused by radiation or chemotherapeutic agents. As for cortisone, while it has the unfortunate property of being immunosuppressive, it is sometimes useful in combating inflammation, fatigue, or depression. Furthermore, it has produced brilliant results in certain leukemias and has had significant effects on breast cancers.

When judiciously employed, hormones are only slightly or very slightly toxic. There are some specific conditions in which they are very valuable, others in which their use is more debatable. Hormone therapy has never met with the vehement opposition that chemotherapy arouses in surgeons and radiotherapists. To many it represents the intellectual model of the ideal therapy: selective, inhibiting only the growth of the target tissue. Things are not that simple, but it is clear that it would be criminal to reject a weapon that can in certain cases halt the development of a tumor, even if only temporarily. The real problem is how to make the best use of it. How can it be perfected? That is the question being asked today by the biochemists who specialize in endocrinology. A recent British publication shows that it is possible to distinguish at least seven different profiles of response of breast cancers to hormones, by making cultures of tumor cells in the presence of various ovarian or pituitary hormones. This requires a technology that is not yet within the reach of every research laboratory, let alone of institutions for the care of patients. But in medicine things generally move quickly, because there is strong pressure for progress, and we can expect to see in the near future very interesting developments in the field of cancer endocrinology. This will make it possible to gain time and spare the patient suffering in a case like the following.

A woman of fifty-five was referred to us with disseminated bone lesions secondary to a breast cancer. After two months of anti-estrogens, there was no improvement. Chemotherapy effectively reduced pain but had only a temporary action. We tried other agents which proved ineffective and had considerable side effects. At the end of six months, having run out of ideas, I prescribed progesterone, without much conviction because statistically the results are disappointing. There was a profound transformation: the disappearance of pain, a weight gain, a return of mobility, and gratitude. As soon as there is a simple test that will enable our colleagues, the endocrinologists, to predict such an individual response, we will rely on it heavily. Until then, we have no choice but to maintain an empirical approach and not become discouraged.

Part Three

❀ ❀ ❀

MODERN WEAPONS

Chemotherapy and immunotherapy, techniques that are in the ferment of rapid development, are much less readily accepted by doctors who are not specialists in cancer than other treatments. But these are techniques that are going to change everything, and they have already begun to do so.

Hormone therapy is an intelligent weapon because it aims at a precise cell. But it is effective only on cancers that are hormone-sensitive, and those are a minority. Radiation, unless it is applied to the entire body—which in small doses is not very effective and in effective doses is lethal—remains a localized weapon, like surgery. If, therefore, we want to eradicate the invisible, disseminated disease, we must turn to other means. Either we must kill the malignant cells wherever they exist—this is the object of cytostatic chemotherapy; or we must raise the level of the body's immunologic defenses, which are inactive or have been overwhelmed—this is the task assigned to immunotherapy.

These weapons will someday be so effective that they will completely transform the treatment of cancer, as chemotherapy has already revolutionized the treatment of acute leukemia in children. At the present time, despite almost daily advances, these techniques alone are usually incapable of curing disseminated cancers. But that is not always true:

more and more cancers are being cured by medical treatments alone. Furthermore, when they are combined with conventional treatments, the results of the latter are notably improved. Finally, there are advances within our reach that might already have been achieved, if the reluctance of many physicians, and of the patients whom they influence, had not prevented certain working hypotheses from being tested.

9

❀❀❀

The Chemotherapies

Here we come to a crucial turning point. The mere word "chemotherapy" causes an attack of gastric acidity and a sudden rise in blood pressure in many physicians who consider it a dangerous—nay, diabolical—weapon and who in spite of the mounting accumulation of facts deny its effectiveness and the progress it has made. I must admit that twenty years ago, the very idea that medicine administered by injections or through the mouth could someday kill cancer cells seemed utterly fantastic. I must also admit that, ten years ago the drugs available were not very effective and the methods of administration were dangerous. Nevertheless, since that time medical opinion has agreed that chemical, synthetic drugs can be effective in the treatment of leukemia, the "liquid" cancer (which is only a cancer of the particular tissue, bone marrow). But medical opinion finds it difficult to accept the fact that "everyday" cancers—tumors of the breast, stomach, lung, and so forth—are susceptible to those same drugs or to others. This is a curious reluctance that is not based solely on scientific considerations.

Fortunately, there have been men and women in every country who don't suffer from such inhibitions and who have set themselves the task of exploring together, in animals and in human patients, the possibilities of these products, which are called "cytostatics" because they are able to arrest the development of cells. There are in the world today thousands of specialists, hundreds of laboratories, and hundreds of specialized treatment centers. Dozens of articles reporting the results of anticancer chemotherapies appear every day in specialized journals around the world, and the body of knowledge built up by the chemotherapists is highly impressive. Moreover, it is their work that has given birth to the new discipline of cell kinetics, and that has been the basis for many new discoveries in physiology which are used in hematology, in immunology, in the chemotherapy of organ transplants, and even in cell biology.

In this chapter I will try to show where chemotherapy stands today, what problems it encounters, and along what lines it will probably develop. The description of its methodology may be of some interest to nonspecialists. An entire discipline has had to be created—in twenty years we have gone from the first crude observations to refined, predictive mathematical models—and the community of chemotherapists takes a certain pride in the work it has accomplished.

In 1934, List and Dustin discovered, on an entirely empirical basis, that colchicine, which had long been used successfully in the treatment of gout, was an antimitotic—that is, that in the cell cycle it blocked mitosis, or the division into two daughter cells. In 1940, S. A. Waksman, who was to receive the Nobel Prize in 1952 for his discovery of streptomycin, the first antituberculosis drug, discovered actinomycin, an antimitotic derived from a mushroom, whose anticancer properties were to be recognized a few years later. In 1943 a Liberty ship, the *John E. Harvey,* sank with a hundred tons of mustard gas aboard, and this catastrophe caused a decrease in the leukocytes of the seamen survivors, an anomaly described by a Navy doctor, Peter Alexander. His report attracted the attention of laboratory researchers, who noted that substances that cause a reduction in the number of leukocytes have destructive effects on experimental tumors, because they inhibit synthesis of the various proteins in all cells that are dividing, blood cells or tumor cells. Since leukocytes, like cancer cells, are in constant proliferation, it is very likely that a substance that blocks the multiplication of the one will have a similar effect on the other.

Researchers lost no time in trying to extract an injectable compound from mustard gas. They succeeded. The first trials with human beings were conducted in 1946. The product has been improved since, but it still exists. It is the first cytostatic of the alkylating class, a series of very effective agents. The inhibiting effect on tumors of another substance toxic for leukocytes, urethane, was also discovered in 1946. In 1947, Sidney Farber produced the first remissions in acute childhood leukemia by the use of aminopterin, a cytostatic whose direct descendant, obtained by biochemists, remains one of the most effective on solid tumors as well as on leukemias. Since then, hardly a year has passed without the introduction of new anticancer chemical compounds, some derived by the chemical manipulation of an existing compound, some the first members of an entirely new family of substances.

The biochemists who specialize in the study of cytostatics are sometimes ahead of the physicians (as when they synthesize a substance that, in view of the effect it can have on cell metabolism, they think might have anticancer properties) and sometimes behind them (as when they exhaust themselves studying a compound the experimenters have already found to be effective, trying—not always successfully—to discover just how it works).

They have been able to identify some substances that attack one or both helixes of DNA by creating a biochemical lesion called an alkylation, and others that destroy some of the RNAs or inhibit RNA polymerase, an enzyme that governs the building of its strands. Certain compounds block cellular division itself. Others are antimetabolites: made to resemble the intermediary products necessary for the building of DNA, RNA, or certain indispensable proteins, they deceive the cell and take the place of those products, with the result that nonviable compounds are formed. The mechanism that controls many active compounds now in use—like the nitrosoureas—is very imperfectly understood. They are active in animals and in human beings, but we don't yet know why. It is already easy to see, however, how much their use helps advance our knowledge of the biochemistry of both normal cells and cancer cells, and how important these studies are for the future progress of chemotherapy.

The elucidation of the relationship between the structure and function of the cytostatics is a discipline that absorbs a great deal of money at present, but the investment is worthwhile. It has already led to the improvement of many substances that were largely ineffective or too toxic, and to the elaboration of new products that are of the greatest interest.

Nevertheless, cancer chemotherapy is still far from being a royal road. One important obstacle in the path is the difficulty of delivering a sufficient concentration of biologically active products wherever the cancer cells are located. Any substance that is suddenly injected into the body is diluted in the bloodstream, and the amount that reaches a given area is small. The amount also depends on the degree of local vascularization (this makes it particularly difficult to introduce cytostatics into areas that have already been irradiated). In addition, the drug is immediately subject to processes of elimination—urinary and digestive—and of transformation and detoxification. Consequently, an active compound's "half-life" in the blood—that is, the time it takes for its concentration to diminish by half—is sometimes very short, on the order of half an hour. This disadvantage can be counteracted by increasing the dose injected or by replacing a sudden injection by a more or less lengthy perfusion. It is clear that in that case we lose in toxicity what we gain in effectiveness. Indeed, the whole recent history of cancer chemotherapy can be summed up in the search for the best possible compromise between those two effects, and we shall see that some very original solutions have been found.

The sensitivity of different phases to chemotherapy follows the same pattern as that for radiotherapy. Certain chemotherapeutic agents are active on only one phase of the cell cycle, or even on only one portion of a given phase. Under these conditions, not only does a product act for only a limited time, but even during that time it acts on only a limited number of cells, while the others continue to thrive with impunity. There are other products that act on all phases of the cycle of division, which represents a much higher biological return, or at any rate on two or more different phases. The problem of finding agents that are active on cells during the rest phase—G_0 or very prolonged G_1 —has so far defied solution.

The resistance of mutant cells is a complex phenomenon of the greatest importance, and it has already been the subject of a multitude of experimental studies that have produced some fascinating biochemical results. To put it briefly, if we consider a billion individuals of any species, whether they be men or grains of wheat, we can't count on their all being biologically identical. In fact, we find the contrary. If we take the case of tubercle bacilli, one out of a million continues to develop in the presence of isoniazid, which kills all the others. This single bacillus is equipped with metabolic circuits that enable it to synthesize in unusual ways the indispensable substances whose synthesis is blocked by isoniazid in susceptible bacilli. The means by which cancer cells resist cytostatics are very varied, and a great many of them have been clearly identified: presence of enzymes that destroy the drug, or reduced permeability of the cell membrane for the agent, or a "short-circuit" analogous to that of the tubercle bacillus, and so forth. There is also a mechanism identical to the one through which the cell resists ionizing radiation: the existence of enzymes capable of "repairing" DNA that has been damaged by an alkylation. That is why in chemotherapy as in radiotherapy we sometimes see a temporary "cytostasis" followed by resumed proliferation; or on the contrary, we may observe delayed cell death that occurs after from two to four generations and is due to imperfect repair of the biochemical lesions caused by a single brief contact with the drug.

In order to establish the objectives and modalities of a course of chemotherapy, it is obviously crucial to ask what the resistance rate of a given tumor is for a given cytostatic. This is a question that is very difficult to answer, and experimental studies are of little help here because they deal with tumors that have been "domesticated" by transmission through a series of animals or induced in selected animals by carcinogenic agents. Spontaneous tumors in human beings are said to be polyclonal—that is, they are usually composed of cell populations that are genetically heterogeneous, of mutants, and we would therefore expect to find a large number of individuals differing from the norm. This is in fact the case. Together with Michel Duchatellier, a young physicist who did his doctoral thesis in my unit, and my student and friend Philippe Chahinian, who is now in New York, I have tried to work out a mathematical model for evaluating the resistance of human tumors to the commonest cytostatic agents. (This study, which is still in progress, is being carried out under a five-year grant from the Health Insurance Fund for the Region of Paris that was awarded at the request of the National Institute of Health and Medical Research.) Our preliminary results, which of course are only approximate, are somewhat dismaying, since they show that the average resistance is between 1 percent and 1 per 1,000. That means that out of a tumor having 10^{11} cells (considerable but not massive size), a very good cytostatic agent used in the best possible way will leave alive 10^8 cells, which will imperturbably go on proliferating. It will take them ten doublings to reconstitute a capital of 10^{11} cells, all of them resistant. If the rate of resistance was 1 percent, scarcely more than six doublings would be required. Those are the facts that therapists must meditate on if they want to plan effective offensive strategies.

As a lung specialist, I can't resist recalling in this connection the beginnings of tuberculosis chemotherapy, between 1947 and 1952. Streptomycin alone killed 9,999 bacilli out of 10,000. It was not enough. Para-aminosalicylic acid killed only 99 bacilli out of 100. Alone, it too was ineffective. But a combination of the two drugs brought about the first cures even before the advent of isoniazid. Classifying cytostatics by order of increasing number of resistant cells encountered in a given tumor gives a very accurate picture of their relative therapeutic value.

The limitations due to cell kinetics are also very important, and for a long time they weren't understood. Yet my great friend Abraham Goldin of the National Cancer Institute—that quiet American who turns up at every decisive crossroad of experimental chemotherapy—had long since demonstrated that methotrexate could cure mice inoculated with L1210 leukemia if the inoculum was weak—or if they were treated early, which comes to the same thing—while it failed when the number of cells had risen beyond a certain threshold. Other Americans, Skipper and Schabel, have made a thorough study of this phenomenon and have expressed it in mathematical terms. What are the reasons for this? One, which I think these authors have somewhat underestimated, relates simply to the resistance rate we have just been talking about. The probability that resistant mutants will appear increases with the number of individual cells. Another reason, and a primary one, is that the larger a tumor becomes, the greater the number of cells that are not engaged in the proliferation cycle, the cells in phase G_0, and hence the smaller the proportion of cells that are potentially vulnerable to chemotherapy. The "coefficient of proliferation," which can be between 90 and 95 percent for foci of a few thousand cells, drops to 10 percent or less for tumors large enough to be palpable; and of course for conventional chemotherapy this represents a seemingly insurmountable obstacle.

But why is this so? It appears that the farther tumor cells are from the center, the fewer the nutrients they receive and therefore the lower their metabolism is. This slowing down might reach a point of almost total quiescence, a cessation of metabolic exchanges, and naturally that would nullify any chemical attack. If a poison proved toxic only during periods of violent muscular effort, men asleep would show no sensitivity to it. Perhaps there are other reasons as well? In any event, the phenomenon is of the utmost importance. We shall have to give further thought to its implications, for it clearly means that a chemotherapeutic attack is most effective when it is used early, against small —even microscopic—tumors.

The lowering of immunity is only one aspect of the toxicity of chemotherapies, a subject we will take up next. Most of the cytostatics diminish immune response by blocking the proliferation of the leukocytes responsible for them. The result may be not only to facilitate the growth of the tumor but also, of course, to facilitate infections— microbial, viral, or fungal—like those that are observed in patients with heart or kidney transplants. Still, we should not overestimate this negative effect: it must be remembered that the cancer itself, if it is large, will already have weakened the immunologic defenses to a great extent, and may even have completely destroyed them.

The undeniable toxicity of chemotherapeutic agents is attributable to the fact that they are still almost totally nonselective, being picked up not by cancer cells in particular but by all the tissues that proliferate fastest. These include the bone marrow (which manufactures leukocytes, red corpuscles, platelets), the digestive tract (which is responsible in particular for assimilating everything the body needs for a normal state of nutrition), the scalp, the skin, and certain endocrine glands. In addition, for unknown reasons, most of the cytostatics can bring on nausea or vomiting. The reader can readily imagine, therefore, that if they are employed without discernment, as they were fifteen years ago, the cytostatics are veritable poisons, acute or chronic, that add immensely to the discomfort and suffering of patients in exchange for a dubious improvement. Between 1962 and 1964, in cases of advanced lung cancer, I myself tried various chemotherapies, which proved disappointing because of their toxicity, could be administered only in a hospital setting, and could by no means be continued as long as necessary. But to reject chemotherapy today on the basis of its toxicity fifteen years ago is rather like rejecting surgery on the basis of the sixteenth-century statistics of Ambroise Paré. Why is it that instead of capitulating before this accumulation of difficulties, chemotherapists have persevered?

Because chemotherapy has in its favor one theoretical advantage that is of paramount importance. The cytostatics, whether they are injected or ingested, distribute themselves throughout the entire organism, including the most distant sites. If we set aside hormones, which, as we have seen, have equally wide scope but limited effectiveness, the cytostatics are the first really general treatment of the disease of cancer, the first means of reaching—of controlling or preventing—lesions that are spread throughout the organism. Through them we can have an effect not only on the visible metastases, which are often too numerous or too awkwardly placed to be cut out or irradiated, but also and especially on the invisible ones, which are almost always present and which represent the chief danger in the medium-range future when a tumor has been operated on or irradiated.

So great is this advantage that thousands of specialists in experimental and clinical chemotherapy have been trying for years to exploit it to best advantage by seeking ways to circumvent the many obstacles I have described. Certain solutions were devised ten years ago, others are recent, and others are still being worked out.

This second-generation chemotherapy is already practiced in centers and units where doctors are well informed—and well taught. Unfortunately, first-generation chemotherapy is still too often practiced by physicians and surgeons who are not up-to-date. The doses prescribed are inadequate, so that they are ineffective in addition to being toxic, and thus, through ignorance, is perpetuated the myth that chemotherapy is worthless as well as intolerable.

When Abraham Goldin discovered that if methotrexate was administered only once every four days, it cured many more mice of leukemia L1210 than if the same total amount was broken down into four daily doses, it was a giant step forward conceptually. That meant that the way in which a given dose of a cytostatic was divided over a period of time could be very important tactically, because it changed the relationship between effectiveness and toxicity. In reality, daily administration—which was the rule with patients only ten years ago, simply because it made a convenient routine and because most other diseases were treated so—did more damage to the organism than to the tumor. Therefore it was necessary to find the optimal schedule for administration of each drug, on the basis of the rate of speed at which it was used by the tumor and by the bone marrow.

I hardly need say that this optimal schedule has not yet been determined for every tumor and every cytostatic. But it is already indisputably established that intermittent administration, ranging from every week to every six weeks according to the situation, is much less toxic and yet provides much better therapeutic results, in particular by exploiting the differences in the speed of regeneration of the tumor and of normal tissues. Thus, intermittent treatments cause more than merely a temporary lowering of immunity; they also stimulate an immunologic "rebound" that sometimes exceeds the initial level and is certainly beneficial, as was shown by my colleague and friend Evan Hersch of Houston, Texas. A corollary to this advantage is that it is possible to avoid various infections, as well as excessive lowering of the number of red and white blood cells, weight loss, digestive disturbances, and so forth. Most of our patients live at home while they are being treated. Many go to work. Progress is undeniable. Not a week passes at Lariboisière without our receiving patients whom enthusiastic but ill-informed doctors have subjected to daily chemotherapies. By changing to semi-monthly or sometimes monthly treatments, we instantly change the effectiveness/toxicity ratio to the patient's advantage.

In 1965, when I published my first attempts to treat disseminated cancers by a combination of five drugs not having "cross resistance" to each other, I was violently criticized by several colleagues. Some told me that it was too toxic, others that it was useless. They were wrong and I was right, as events were to prove. Min C. Li, in 1960, and Ezra Greenspan of the Mount Sinai School of Medicine of the City University of New York, in 1962, had already combined cytostatics. The combinations were promising and eventually revealed themselves to be superior to the "monotherapies" they have since replaced. But I didn't know about their work, and neither did those who contradicted me, apparently.

On the theoretical level, the idea of combining drugs was unassailable. It was suggested to me by the situation with regard to tuberculosis, which was still a very difficult disease at the time. In tuberculosis, everything might be lost if drugs were given consecutively, whereas everything was won if they were given simultaneously. At that time, the tuberculosis specialists were finding out that it was criminal not to combine various drugs, because in administering them consecutively they were creating by selection resistant strains that killed the patients. Yet in the same wards where pulmonary tuberculosis patients were being treated with a combination of three drugs having different mechanisms of action and no "cross resistance," lung-cancer patients were still being given a single cytostatic. This inconsistency suddenly became obvious to me in 1963, and that was how I first became interested in cancer. Today one has only to open the *Cancer Treatment Reports* published regularly by the U.S. National Cancer Institute to realize that ten years later, the cause of polychemotherapies has definitely triumphed—among the professionals, if not among the amateurs.

In deference to truth, I must point out that in France, shortly before I began defending the use of combined chemotherapies for cancer, Claude Jacquillat of Jean Bernard's team in Paris, and Claude Dargent and Marcel Pommateau in Lyons, had already begun to fight for simultaneous use of several cytostatics. Also, the hematologists had been convinced for some time that the progress they were making against leukemia was due to increasingly rich combinations. Today, although oncologists disagree about the details, the great majority of them recognize the principle and have forgotten how fiercely they opposed it. When someone introduces an innovation, people call him a dangerous madman. Later they declare that the innovation is not mad, but it is unimportant. In the end, they say it is very important, but of course everyone has known about it for a long time.

Here again, it goes without saying that we can and must refine, and that not every combination is necessarily an improvement. There are even some combinations of drugs that have proved to be less effective than one of them used alone. Nonetheless, the concept is fundamental. A few figures will enable the reader to judge:

If a large tumor contains 10^{12} cells, and if the rate of resistance to a cytostatic is 1 percent, or 10^{-2}, by combining five active drugs that do not counteract each other, we leave alive only 100 cells. But in ten doublings they will again reach 100,000, and in twenty doublings 100,000,000. And since, as we have seen, the rate of growth of a tumor decreases regularly, the doubling time is much shorter when there are 100,000 cells than when there are 100,000,000, so that the time gained is less than one might think. Above all, it is clear that even if intensive chemotherapy is used, it is impossible to eradicate a very large tumor. If, therefore, one decided to make the number of drugs to be combined proportionate to the apparent size of the tumor, one would be committing a serious error. The "heavy" chemotherapies are today a means of eradicating tumors of moderate size. By the same token, the argument sometimes advanced by certain oncologists who are not chemotherapists, that chemotherapy should be "reserved" for the time when metastases become palpable and begin to grow perceptibly, is absolutely illogical. It is the embodiment of both ignorance and defeatism. Treatment must always be instituted as soon as possible. With solid tumors, it is never a matter of days, but it may be a matter of weeks.

The evaluation of chemotherapies presents a surprising paradox. Their results are still calculated on large tumors, while we have just seen that they act much better on tumors of very small volume. Basically, that is because for a long time instead of studying chemotherapies as complements to surgery or radiotherapy, the chemotherapists let themselves be affected by the hostile environment in which they worked and treated only desperate cases, those that their colleagues were willing to abandon to them. That was already a vicious circle, since the poor results they obtained were an argument for not entrusting them with "good" cases. In 1952, when isoniazid revealed its astonishing anti-tuberculosis properties, my teacher Etienne Bernard remarked that if it had been tried on cases of inveterate, extensive tuberculosis, it would have been declared of no great value. In any event, as a protection against their own possible overenthusiasm, the chemotherapists decided to count as a partial response only a diminution of more than 50 percent in the mathematical product of two perpendicular diameters of a well-circumscribed lesion, without increase in, or appearance of, another lesion in the meantime, and to consider any lesser result as a failure. Complete responses need no definition. The duration of a response is the time between the obtaining of the minimal partial response and a regrowth of more than 25 percent based on the lowest point reached. By adopting these rules, the chemotherapists were able to define the various cytostatics by the rate of response they produced in a given tumor and the distribution of the durations of response. One very important point is that the duration of survival of patients who respond favorably to the treatment is usually very long compared to the duration of survival in cases of failure. If 10 percent of the cases subject to a given chemotherapy respond, the rate is low. It is nonetheless true that the average length of survival of the patients who do respond is four or five times greater than that of the subjects who don't react to the treatment in accordance with the definition and six or eight times that of the subjects who aren't treated at all. That is a strong argument for trying a chemotherapy in all cases, even if we know that the rate of response to it is low, on the understanding that it can quickly be stopped or changed for patients whom it doesn't benefit. Since, as we have demonstrated at Lariboisière, the response is always obtained in the first six weeks, with an experienced chemotherapist there is no risk of uselessly prolonging an ineffective treatment.

The results given below relate to advanced, disseminated cancers that were immediately judged to be beyond the resources of both surgery and radiotherapy. They were obtained, up until 1972–73, with intermittent polychemotherapies of an empirical nature, and are given as an illustration of what was possible a few years ago. Published by various international teams, these results are not controversial, and if anything, are minimized by comparison with the results of the latest studies.

In disseminated breast cancers, the rate of response varies from 40 to 80 percent depending on the combinations used. After the work of

Greenspan, then Cooper in the United States, it suddenly became apparent that even in cases of dissemination, breast cancers were so sensitive to combined chemotherapies that their prognosis had been transformed. That fact is not yet well enough known, and we receive many desperate cases that have been referred to us by the nth doctor consulted, after many others have for months advised abstention from treatment. Even then, we observe a high percentage of very favorable results. By this I mean the regression of metastases of the liver or bone, cases of women who were pinned to their beds by pain able to walk again and resume an almost normal life. Of course there are failures. The doctors who are waiting for us to cure 100 percent of cases before they deign to take an interest in chemotherapy are still legion. But it is extraordinary, fascinating, wonderful, to note that there are successes. Several dozens of our patients who are in ambulatory treatment today were bedridden one or two years ago. And these are results that can be reproduced by everyone; there is no mystery about them.

Moreover, they have already been exceeded by the third-generation treatments I shall discuss below. Of course, even in cases of success, no one yet dares speak of permanent cure, least of all myself. We maintain constant therapeutic pressure, calling upon all our powers of persuasion, because our patients, ready for anything in the beginning, quickly forget the state they were in and want nothing so much as to stop a treatment that, even if it is acceptable compared to their former symptoms, is still a burden to them. But we dare not stop. We are waiting for the recurrences that, statistically, must someday appear in some of them.

But here too there is something new and striking: we no longer await them with a fatalistic attitude. A cytostatic developed in Italy a few years ago, which has no cross resistance with the combination of drugs generally used first, has shown that in at least a third of the cases that do not respond to that combination, it can induce sizable regressions. In short, in the last few years, disseminated breast cancer has entered the ranks of cancers that can be controlled and perhaps cured. That makes it even more important to administer treatment early. Even cases that only recently were still given up for lost can be transformed. How are we to get that message across to the great Parisian lung specialist who, observing pulmonary metastases appearing four years after surgical removal of a breast cancer, ordered laboratory tests for tubercle bacilli so as to "gain time" and prescribed trivial treatments for the patient's "psychological comfort," while she, meantime, found it increasingly hard to breathe? I saw this patient in the hospital four months late, at the insistence of her family. We instituted a treatment that worked, as I was sure it would. It is still too early to tell much. The patient can breathe. I have one more enemy.

In metastasized cancers of the colon, the rate of response varies, according to combinations and teams, from 15 to 30 percent. The use of new cytostatics has just made it possible to pass the 30 percent figure, which for a long time no one had been able to better.

A patient was sent to us eighteen months ago for an enormous abdominal tumor that had recurred after surgery. It was impossible to operate upon and unresponsive to radiation. The surgeon who referred the patient to us does not yet belong to the band of those who think that systematic postoperative chemotherapy would be more effective. But he is already one of those who think that in the case of an extensive recurrence, it is not a crime to try chemotherapy. This patient, who is receiving weekly ambulatory treatment, is better. We have obtained a partial regression, which is being stabilized by continued treatment and which makes it possible for him to lead a family and social life. Our patient is fighting to maintain that regression. He knows what is at stake. We would have preferred to see him earlier. But we know that if we had received him in the same condition two or three years ago, we could not have done so much for him. He knows it too, and he knows that other drugs, even more active, will come.

This is not the same situation as with breast cancers, but we do not understand the reasons for the differences. At present it is better to have a hepatic metastasis that comes from a cancer of the breast than one that comes from a cancer of the colon. It is nevertheless undeniable that a third of the cases formerly beyond our reach now respond to treatment. Charles G. Moertel of the Mayo Clinic team devotes himself almost exclusively to the treatment of these cases, and in a few years has given us chemotherapeutic weapons and strategies that have changed the situation. That is what counts. Wherever a breach is opened, the chemotherapists rush in, try a hundred variations on the same theme, add drugs, modify doses, adjust time lapses, change methods of administration—and advance. I am physically tired from almost monthly trips to the United States or elsewhere, where in two days we communicate to each other our observations on the latest improvements that have been thought up in this daily battle. But there is hardly a trip from which I don't return with some small, encouraging innovation, some slight advance, or some project based on an interesting observation.

Disseminated lung cancers are even more resistant to our chemotherapies today than intestinal cancers, to the point where many doctors advise morphine alone and consider attempts at treatment in these situations to be experimentation, pure and simple. Yet for one of the most serious varieties, which has proved very sensitive, we have already reached a rate of response of 80 percent. For the others, we are approaching 50 percent, an enormous result, considering what we knew only three years back. Unfortunately the duration of response is shorter than for other cancers. In any event, these results, though modest, are already such that I fail to understand how one can justify abstaining from treatment. Once again, not to persist in a treatment that has proven ineffective is the least evidence of wisdom one should expect of a physician. But not to try it when it might succeed is inexcusable, even if one knows that under the best of circumstances, the end will be only palliation and not cure. After all, many chronic diseases, including some that are very severe, are today given palliative treatments without arousing anyone's indignation. It would be considered a crime —and rightly so—not to treat certain cases of cardiac insufficiency on the ground that we can only attenuate them and prolong their course. The vehement intransigence of certain doctors who want their cancer patients to have a complete recovery or nothing is something that never ceases to amaze me.

A patient came to see us on his own in 1971. He knew that he had a severe, diffuse variety of lung cancer. The provincial cancer clinic where he was being treated without success had warned his family that they must abandon hope. Today this patient is free from any detectable lesion and for the last few months has been undergoing only light treatment. I recently presented him to a specialist in New York at Memorial Hospital, where nothing much surprises them any more, and for once my colleague abandoned his customary imperturbability. But there is nothing astonishing about these cases. We have other patients who are only six or twelve months behind this one. And yet recently the family doctor said to the husband of a patient of mine who had been transformed by six months of chemotherapy and was once again fit and smiling, "What's the point?"

A short time ago I presented my results to a very Parisian scientific society, and a well-known lung specialist—who also uses chemotherapy on his cancer patients and who wishes me well, incidentally—expressed surprise at the difference between the number of our successes and his. It happens that he specializes in the treatment of certain serious pulmonary diseases, which nothing in the world would persuade me to treat myself because my experience of them is only second-hand and much inferior to his. One day the statisticians in the United States discovered that the rate of complete remissions of acute childhood leukemia was much higher in the hematology departments than in the general pediatric wards. That settled the question, and in the United States cancers are treated by cancer specialists. Still, I must amend that statement. If the American Society of Clinical Oncology asked me, at its meeting of May 1976, to chair the session devoted to lung cancers, it was not only because I have been obtaining good results, but also because I am a lung specialist, and perhaps the latter partly explains the former. It is certain that the future belongs to subspecializations and redistributions of competence. It is better for bronchial cancers to be treated by oncologists who know what a lung is, or by lung specialists who have a good background in oncology, than by general chemotherapists. It may be unimportant for the treatment of breast tumors, but not for the treatment of certain organs that have complex and critical functions.

The most interesting aspect of chemotherapy is its aspect as a science-in-the-making. I want to take a brief look at the third generation of chemotherapeutic tactics so as to give the reader an idea of the nature and scope of the research in which applied scientists the world over are currently engaged.

As in radiotherapy, the concept of synchronization is very attractive. Many regimens are being tried in an attempt to use drug A to synchronize large fractions of cell populations as they pass through the cycle so as to increase the number of those that, at a given moment, will be simultaneously in a phase sensitive to drug B. Progress in this area is slow, but experiments indicate that it will be a fruitful avenue of research. There is still the danger of also synchronizing the cells of the bone marrow or digestive tract and hence of increasing toxicity. Further studies of cell kinetics may enable us to take optimum advantage of the differences in length of cycle of normal cells and cancer cells.

Cells that remain in phase G_0 and hence do not proliferate are insensitive or only slightly sensitive to drugs. Is it possible to make them join the proliferating contingent? In the days following the administration of a strong dose of an agent that is active on all phases of the cycle, the tumor may be so depleted and the vascularization so improved that quiescent cells, finding more favorable conditions, again start proliferating and thus become sensitive to an agent that is active on a particular phase of the cycle. This is true experimentally, as Skipper and Schabel have shown, providing the timing is exact. It may be true clinically. Many teams are currently trying to demonstrate it. Any success in this field would quickly have enormous repercussions, as it would make chemotherapies effective in situations where they are still powerless.

A kind of shock wave ran through the community of chemotherapists not long ago when Sutherland of Great Britain showed that metronidazole, which I have already mentioned in connection with radiotherapy, not only sensitized cells to radiation but, independently of radiation, could also kill cells in phase G_0—a result that is yet to be confirmed but the possible significance of which can be readily imagined. If that is true, it will of course be necessary to study the effect of this product on the stem cells of bone marrow, because the cell reserves, which are in G_0 in the marrow, play an exceedingly important role throughout life, and it would be very dangerous to destroy them. We are awaiting further results, which should be available shortly. It was again Goldin who observed a few years ago that while very strong doses of a certain cytostatic were toxic for the host as well as for the tumor, the simultaneous administration of its antidote eliminated both the toxicity and the anticancer effect. He then began looking for the optimal interval for administration of the two agents, which would enable him to inundate the organism with massive doses of the drug and to use the antidote to "rescue" the bone marrow without diminishing the anticancer effect. The time interval, he discovered, should be a few hours.

This method, applied in the United States by Isaac Djerassi to leukemias and lung cancers, and by Norman Jaffe and Emil Frei III to osteosarcomas, was introduced into France by Georges Mathé. Extraordinary results have been published by Jaffe and Frei of Children's Hospital in Boston in the treatment of pulmonary metastases of osteosarcomas in adolescents. I shall come back to this later in connection with postoperative chemotherapy. At present, several teams are trying to develop this model of rescue, and some fascinating results have already been reported by the Boston team, following a change of antidote.

What emerges from these studies is that by the rescue technique one can safely apply nearly a hundred times the dose of cytostatic that would otherwise be considered a maximum, and with perhaps ten times greater benefit. In other words, for a leading cytostatic agent, we have already discovered a technique that makes it possible to multiply its effectiveness by ten without increasing its toxicity. This discovery reflects a mixture of theroretical thinking and ingenious exploitation of present possibilities which accurately reflects the frame of mind of those who are engaged in research on the treatment of cancer. It happens that as I write these lines one of my patients is in Boston, where I sent him for a treatment with which I am not familiar, and which calls for the rapid administration of a dose equal to two hundred times the usual dose. Tolerance is good, the immediate effect astounding. Frei reports that some of his patients have already received five hundred doses at a time.

But it is not enough for the cytostatic to circulate. It must enter the cells to make lesions in them. Certain cancer cells resist penetration, but biochemical manipulation might make them more accessible. Substances as nontoxic as chlorpromazine, theophylline, and vitamin A have accomplished this experimentally. They are now being tested in human beings. Here chemotherapy reaches a degree of refinement, without additional toxicity, that demands the talents of an engineer more than those of a scientist. There is a problem: the imperfect permeability of the membrane of certain cells to given molecules. There is therefore a solution, somewhere. Thanks to the close and constant communication that exists today between clinical and experimental chemotherapists, the doctor's request is heard, the problem he has formulated is taken up by the appropriate experimenter. We can imagine the "fallout" there may be for the fundamental study of the physiology of cell membranes. The problem of the existence of anti-ligases is another "simple" question of engineering. If we could somehow inhibit the enzymes that repair the damage induced in DNA by certain cytostatics, what an advantage it would be! The whole contingent of cells that recuperate would be struck dead by a single dose of the toxic product. At a recent International Congress of Chemotherapy (London, 1975), it was rumored that, as I have already suggested, caffeine had such a property. This is not the place to explain why that is plausible from a biochemical point of view. Let us wait for confirmation. In any event, it is certain that one day we will have "anti-repair" measures at our disposal. As soon as that happens, without any increase in toxicity, the effectiveness of chemotherapies will be multiplied by a factor of three, four, or five.

Treatment protocols generally provide fixed lengths of time between two consecutive treatments, but that is only a matter of intellectual laziness. Together with Duchatellier and Chahinian, I have shown that the best mathematical model of response to treatment is one that provides a minimum of four treatments per doubling time. In other words, it is possible and desirable to individualize therapy on the basis of the tumor's rate of growth. We are trying to convince our American friends to test this hypothesis in the field, which presents some practical difficulties. But it is clear that oncologists will soon come to regard it as completely unjustifiable to treat a tumor that doubles in twenty days in the same way as a tumor that doubles in two hundred. A few cases of our own already confirm this and point to the following conclusion: while a tumor that is developing rapidly can be controlled only by a massive chemotherapy, a tumor that is developing slowly may respond to infinitely less aggressive treatments, administered every four to six weeks, which will not even interfere with the social and professional life of the patient. That is why, before establishing the program for a long-term course of treat-

ment, I think it is crucial to collect as much information as possible
on the rate of growth in an individual case.

The blood of cancer patients contains more fibrin than the blood of
other subjects. Tumors contain a high level of fibrin and thromboplas-
tin, compounds that are necessary to clotting in case of hemorrhage.
Metastases need fibrin in order to develop. To top all these findings—
which obviously represent an impressive series of experimental studies,
which I am not mentioning—an English doctor noticed some ten years
ago that subjects who were given anticoagulants for coronary disease
suffered significantly fewer cancers than a control population of the
comparable age group. I have already spoken about anticoagulants after
surgery. How about anticoagulants during chemotherapy? Might they
be capable of helping the cytostatics to penetrate the tumor? George
Elias in Buffalo, New York, is presently exploring this hypothesis,
which is clearly of great interest. And at Lariboisière, the team of
Jacques Caen—another of Jean Bernard's assistants—and my own
team have just discovered another phenomenon of the same order,
which differentiates the cancer patient from the normal subject and
can be an obstacle to the effect of chemotherapy. We are trying to get
around it. Here again, it is a problem of engineering. We make an
inventory of the practical obstacles to the effect of our drugs. We attack
them one by one. Some have already been overcome. Our results as a
whole show the improvement.

More than one book could be written—and indeed has been written
—about the manipulation of cell resistance. I will mention only one
aspect of it. It has been observed that when a tumor becomes resistant
to a given cytostatic, its sensitivity to another cytostatic may be appre-
ciably increased. For example, tumor cells may acquire metabolic path-
ways with no alternative and so become very vulnerable: if these path-
ways are blocked, the cell dies. This "collateral sensitivity" has already
been successfully exploited experimentally. So far as I know, there has
been no attempt to use it in the treatment of human beings, but I
would be very surprised if such an attempt were not made soon. With
the manipulation of resistance, we are deep into a very sophisticated
biochemistry, but there are plenty of centers equipped to carry out such
research successfully.

•   •   •

After this discussion of scientific efforts—or technical efforts, if the reader prefers—let us examine briefly the concrete conditions under which chemotherapeutic treatments are conducted.

Apart from a few special situations, we administer all our treatments on an outpatient basis. The fact that the treatments have become intermittent makes prolonged presence at the hospital unnecessary in most cases. The patient lives in his family environment, often continues professional activities, and comes to our unit—or is brought to us, as the case may be—for a stay of two hours every seven to twenty-eight days. Chemotherapy is no longer the difficult, toxic treatment it was ten years ago. At any rate, it is less and less so. Clearly, this is to the advantage of society, because, the way we operate it, a treatment unit of five beds renders the same service as a hospital ward of a hundred and fifty beds with a full staff for three eight-hour shifts, hotel equipment, and so forth. But above all, it is to the advantage of the patients. At the first consultation they almost always tell us, "If I can go on living at home, I agree to everything else." I have not yet spoken of oral chemotherapies. Personally, I am watching their development closely. We have perhaps half a score of cytostatics that are very active when administered by mouth, and others that are still at an experimental stage. We are perfecting combinations that, while they meet the most rigorous requirements of modern chemotherapies and give excellent results, can be administered in the form of little pills. This de-dramatization of chemotherapy, which is so important for the patient and also for his family doctor, may help us to conquer the resistance against chemotherapy that persists. Certain indispensable agents that are destroyed by the digestive juices will always have to be injected. But in many situations we will be able to use an entirely oral treatment.

One of our women patients, who has a cancer of the lung with dissemination to the bones and to the opposite lung, has been treated with pills for eighteen months and continues to lead a normal family and professional life. Another, who has a disseminated cancer of the breast, is going into her third year of ambulatory treatment with a combination of drugs administered orally. Dozens of patients who have had perfusions, or who have heard about them, are surprised that they can be treated by pills. Practicing physicians who send us their patients, after warning them of what "lies in store" for them, can't believe their eyes when they read our prescriptions and telephone us. There is a lot going on in this area.

These are the facts I wanted to lay before readers who are not informed about cancer chemotherapy. It is a method of treatment that is effective and indispensable and is the object of much lively research cutting across various disciplines. It is a method that is making very rapid progress.

To dignify by the name of chemotherapy approaches that are clumsy and incompetent, and then, on the ground that they prove unsuccessful, to declare that chemotherapy is a failure, is a piece of glaring— though common—dishonesty. To accuse the chemotherapy of today of the sins of ten years ago, when everything has changed several times over during the intervening period, is an act of unmitigated bad faith. To be sure, chemotherapies do not cure all cancers. They do, however, make possible today results that only yesterday would have seemed like science fiction. And it is obvious to those who practice them correctly and work to improve them that they are raising a rich harvest for tomorrow. The chemotherapists are very much aware of the difficulties they confront. For that very reason, they are organizing to overcome them. The dogs bark, but the caravan moves on.

Throughout this chapter I have tried to show how progress comes about. There are the researchers in the fundamental or semi-fundamental sciences who develop the drugs. There are the experimenters and the therapists who, in fruitful collaboration, close in on the problems posed by the use of those drugs, isolate them, and try to find solutions. I have nothing against pure research or the enormous budgets devoted to it. But I have never perceived more clearly than through my work with cancer how essential it is to have another kind of curiosity as well, a curiosity with an interest at stake—in short, applied research. It is the engineers who have shaped our present society and who are shaping the society of tomorrow. It is the doctors who improve the treatment of the sick. The empiricism that seizes any weapon at hand sometimes succeeds and sometimes fails, thereby raising questions, some of which can be answered empirically, others only by deeper theoretical knowledge. Theoretical knowledge in turn supplies the materials that suddenly help to solve a pending practical problem. It is from this exchange that the progressive increase in our power over nature flows, not from fundamental, theoretical research alone.

Recently my associates and I have been fascinated by the brilliant, rapid, almost unbelievable results of a platinum salt used in pulmonary metastases of certain cancers of the testicle. This agent—the cost of which I don't know, because the U.S. National Cancer Institute sends it to us free—causes the disappearance of enormous lesions that nothing else could touch. It has been "operational" for less than two years, and already we have heard that the NCI's animal experimentation laboratories have new and improved versions of it.

Thus, when we consider the prospects for chemotherapy, we can be almost certain that the next few years will see the emergence of an arsenal of new drugs which—while we will not always understand why they are active (as in the case of platinum)—will be increasingly effective in specific cases and in combination with other agents or other procedures.

10

❀❀❀

Immunotherapy

We now come to the newest of our weapons, one that is even more controversial, if that is possible, than chemotherapy, and one whose basis is by no means certain, or even understood. But it is one that has a very promising future, and some of its results already merit our attention.

In 1958, working separately, Bernard Halpern of the Collège de France, and Lloyd Old, who is now deputy director of the Sloan-Kettering Institute of New York, showed that BCG, the bacillus of L.C.A. Calmette and A.F.M. Guérin, which is used as a tuberculosis vaccine, possesses anticancer properties in animals. At that time it had not yet been demonstrated that cancer cells carry antigens that are different from those of the host and, theoretically, can therefore trigger an immune reaction to destroy and reject them. But in the years following, a succession of uncoordinated attempts were made to use immune reactions to treat tumors. We learned about these reactions in greater detail, there was increasing contact among specialists, and immunotherapy began to emerge from the ghetto where it had at first been confined by—the chemotherapists. Even today it is difficult to give a clear idea of a field that is so indefinite, controversial, and constantly changing. Let me try to do so by examining a few concrete situations in detail and commenting on the results of some attempts to use it. I did not invent immunotherapy for cancer, but I have been so deeply involved in it for so many years that it will be easy for me to refer to my personal adventures.

One beautiful day in 1964, I received from Sir Michael Woodruff, a great surgeon and an even greater immunologist in Edinburgh, a reprint of an article in *Lancet.* In it he reported the beneficial effects he had obtained in advanced cases of cancer by injecting his patients with lymphocytes taken from normal blood donors or from spleens removed from victims of automobile accidents. At that time we did not yet know that there are at least two types of lymphocytes, T and B, and had only imperfect knowledge of the tissue groups discovered by the great French hematologist Jean Dausset. Jacques Delobel, who is now full professor at Amiens, was then a resident in the unit of my teacher, Etienne Bernard, where I was an associate professor. I instructed Delobel to procure a spleen at all costs—that is, to lay siege to the surgeons at Laënnec Hospital. We were promised that afternoon a spleen that was likely to rupture and would have to be removed. Delobel spent several hours in the laboratory under a sterile hood, separating out the lymphocytes as best he could and washing them, and we ended up with a vial that we estimated contained twenty billion viable lymphocytes. I immediately injected them into the abdominal cavity of one of our patients who was dying of a cancer of the ovary that had responded to none of the treatments we had available at the time and who, if she was not to suffocate, had to have eight liters of liquid drawn five times a week from her peritoneum. A miracle: the next day our patient felt better. No further puncture was necessary. Her abdomen dried up. She survived without other treatment for two and a half months, then died suddenly of a cerebral metastasis. Sir Michael's treatment had been temporarily effective. It was based on the hypothesis that for unknown reasons the lymphocytes of cancer patients were inadequate and were no longer able to recognize, or no longer able to reject, the "foreign" cancer cells, and that lymphocytes from normal donors might be able to do so.

Since then, so far as I know, nothing further on the subject has been heard from Edinburgh, because numerous experiments, some of which have been conducted by Sir Michael Woodruff, have shown that matters were much more complicated. But any tangible result fascinated me—and still fascinates me—whatever the explanation for it may be. We immediately started collecting lymphocytes, no longer from the spleens of motor accident victims, but from the blood of normal donors, railroad workers as it happened, who responded to an appeal by our transfusionist, Bernard Gross. And in 1967 we treated seventy patients with disseminated cancers unresponsive to all other therapies with massive injections of circulating lymphocytes, taken from unrelated donors. In one-fourth of the cases we had successes—partial and temporary, but enough to show us that something was going on. I wanted to go further, and instead of extracting our lymphocytes "by hand," to use a blood-cell separator, of which there were two in Paris and a few in the United States. It was too expensive for us. The following year, the women's magazine *Elle* agreed to take up a collection among its readers. The collection brought in a quarter of the sum necessary, and this money was frozen in a bank. I will relate later what became of it, because in the end it was used in the field of immunology. But let us pause here over these lymphocytes. An American, Lawrence, was to show that they contain a "transfer factor" that enables them to transmit their own immunologic memory to "virgin" lymphocytes and to cure certain infections in subjects who have a congenital disease that prevents them from creating their own immunity. This "transfer factor" is used today in the treatment of certain cancers, in particular by a team in San Francisco who report interesting results. My friend Yoseph Pilch of Los Angeles has since gone farther. He has demonstrated that if one immunizes an animal against a tumor, the RNA extracted from the lymphocytes of that animal can also communicate immunity against the same tumor to new animals. Is there therefore a specific "chemical immunologic memory," and could we, for example, extract from the lymphocytes of cured cancer patients a substance that would be useful for the prevention, or even the treatment, of that same type of tumor in others?

It is not impossible. But our donors had never had cancer. Their lymphocytes, therefore, had to stimulate nonspecific immunity. At a time when certain animal experiments were "proving" that such stimulation is impossible and that nonimmune lymphocytes have no effect, other studies showed that Lawrence's factor does exist, but that it is not specific and that it transfers only a general capacity to restore the immunity that the lymphocytes of cancer patients have lost. This sums up the whole story of immunotherapy: a constant avalanche of contradictory results and changing concepts, compared to which the crisis in contemporary physics is the picture of order and harmony. Let us turn, then, to the stimulation of nonspecific immunity, and so come back to BCG.

The discovery of BCG's anticancer properties came as no surprise to the immunologists, who had long been using it, in a complex preparation, to increase immune reactions to various substances. The oncologists rushed into the breach and achieved some successes: Donald Morton with melanomas; Georges Mathé with acute childhood leukemias; Hamilton-Fairley and Powles and many other teams with acute leukemias of adults. Disparate or contradictory results have suggested that there may be differences in the relative effectiveness of the BCG of different countries. The Pasteur Institute has just put on the market a product called "immuno-BCG." David Weiss in Israel has long been exploring an extract of BCG, apparently with some success. For three years the Lung Group of the European Organization has been studying the possibilities of BCG in bronchial cancers. Just recently, two interesting reports were published in *Lancet* showing that BCG had a beneficial effect in such cases either after radiotherapy or, administered by intrapleural route, after surgical removal of the tumor. When applied alone in cases of disseminated tumors, BCG has no effect. On the other hand, it prolongs remission of acute leukemias that have first been treated by chemotherapy, and when it is administered at the same time as a chemotherapy, it reinforces the effects of the latter on several cancers in experimental animals and also in human beings.

Can we explain these facts? Yes, in part, because we know that BCG has the property of "activating" the macrophages and stimulating them to multiply. And activated macrophages do not like tumor cells. When they come into contact with them, they kill them.

Thus a more general problem was raised: was BCG's immunity-stimulating effect the result of a single lucky chance, or was it related to a property common to other families of germs? The second hypothesis proved to be correct. A great many microbes have been capable of stimulating nonspecific immunity. One of them, *Corynebacterium par-*

vum, which has been studied experimentally, especially by Halpern and by Woodruff, is dear to my heart because I have devoted nearly ten years to studying it, and it still holds surprises for me. Injected intravenously (after having been killed by heat), it has proved capable of making very advanced tumors retreat, as has been confirmed by a celebrated team in Houston. It enhances the effects of chemotherapies and significantly prolongs survival in many disseminated cases. And by observing its effects we have been able to attack certain dogmas concerning the conditions of immunotherapy. It is being studied today on a large scale in both America and Europe. There is no doubt in my mind that it has added a new weapon and a new dimension to chemotherapy, although I have the greatest difficulty in persuading the "pure" chemotherapists and immunotherapists to combine their treatments.

There are, then, in nature bacteria that help the organism to rid itself of a cancer. I do not think this is accidental, for the list of such bacteria is too long. The chemical constituents of the membranes of certain microorganisms provoke not only a specific immune response, a "vaccination," but also a reinforcement of the natural defenses against other aggressions. That is probably what has made it possible for complex organisms to survive in an environment dominated by microbes. A vast field is therefore open for investigation.

It is up to us to take advantage of the help that certain bacteria can give us in the fight against cancer, just as, since Sir Alexander Fleming, we have taken advantage of the help that microscopic fungi can give us against bacteria. Many researchers—those at the Pasteur Institute are in the forefront—are trying to identify and purify the molecules responsible for nonspecific immune stimulation. We know a few of these molecules, which act at various levels. It is possible that combining them could lead to poly-immunotherapies, such as we have begun to use empirically with success.

But human intelligence can go further. It can synthesize new agents that stimulate immunity, agents that are more powerful, more refined, or more diversified. Certain laboratories are already doing exactly that. There is no doubt that in time the immunologists and the biochemists will provide us with substances capable of eliminating the strange tolerance of the host organism for the cancer cells it harbors.

Another possibility for immunotherapy consists of trying to increase the power not of the general defense mechanisms but of the specific response to a given tumor. It sometimes happens that the level of a patient's general defenses is good and that he has immune reactions to the antigens of the tumor cells, but that for one reason or another these specific reactions are weak. Many attempts have been made to intensify these reactions by injecting tumor cells at different points in the organism. The cells, taken either from the patient himself (autologous cells) or from a similar case (allogeneic cells), are first killed and treated in various ways to enhance their immunogenic power. This procedure has produced good results in experiments with animals. I myself have had some encouraging results with it in human beings, but the studies in question were uncontrolled and therefore inconclusive.

The first solid results appear to have been obtained by James F. Holland and Bekesi of Mount Sinai Hospital in New York. In a recent study, these investigators used a special process to modify autologous cells and reinjected them into adult leukemia patients. This treatment has enabled patients to survive longer than the group given conventional treatment.

This is a reliable and important contribution to immunotherapy, but we must remember that a new way to treat a disease is not the same thing as a vaccination to prevent it. I do not think it is realistic to expect that we will ever have a vaccination for cancer, because there are so many varieties of the disease that there would have to be hundreds of different vaccines. Nevertheless, we can't rule out the possibility that if it becomes technologically possible, such vaccines may one day be tested for certain high-risk groups—women with a family history of breast cancer, for example.

It is conceivable that we can combine nonspecific stimulation and specific immunization. If we inject BCG into a tumor that is accessible because it is superficial, it is in the hope that the tumor will be destroyed by the influx of activated macrophages that BCG induces. But we may also hope that these macrophages will "learn" from their contact with the tumor cells and transmit the information, provoking an increase in specific immunity such that other lesions, which have not been injected with BCG, will also be destroyed. Certain oncologists have observed results of this sort. Personally, I have tried in vain for five years to reproduce them. That, incidentally, is one of the mysteries of the trade of clinical investigator: why do results vary so considerably from one team to another?

Besides direct attempts to reinforce specific or nonspecific immunity, there is a place in immunotherapy for indirect procedures designed to rid the organism of elements that may impede the normal expression of the immunologic defenses. On the basis of a considerable number of convergent studies, we can now state that the blood of some persons who have tumors contains certain substances that block the specific immunity to tumor cells and others that, in a nonspecific way, block all the immune mechanisms. In other words, tumors manufacture (as Fauve and Jacob have shown) or cause the organism to manufacture (as I myself, along with many others, have shown) substances that protect them from immunologic aggression.

This is where my machine for separating the lymphocytes comes in. (I was finally able to buy it in 1974, thanks to additional gifts.) The idea was, by a series of complex operations, to take the patient's white blood cells, wash them, reinject them along with his red cells, remove his blood plasma containing blocking substances, and replace it with plasma from normal donors. It's easier said than done. I wanted to give this machine to Lariboisière as a gift, but the hospital could not provide me with a place to put it, or funds or personnel to run it. I should point out that a general hospital is not the ideal place to deliver such care and that, indeed, the floor space I needed did not exist. We were able to have the machine installed at the departmental transfusion center in Creteil, a small city southeast of Paris, for the director there is one of my former students. It is now in operation, and our first results are extremely encouraging. Just recently I reported them to a small group in New York, and a renowned immunologist asked me, "Why do you think the improvements you report are due to what you take out and not to what you inject?" A good question. We don't know anything about it, and we are exploring both possibilities by making chemical analyses of the donors' plasma and the patients' plasma, which should suffice to keep us busy for several years. But now that I have observed the initial results, something tells me that we are on the track of some interesting phenomena and that both mechanisms suggested by my American colleague are doubtless at work.

After this somewhat rambling discussion, let us look at some provisional conclusions. Immunotherapy is still in its infancy. Nothing is absolutely certain yet. All the medical oncology teams in the world agree about the results of chemotherapies using alkylating agents, but they fly at one another's throats as soon as anyone mentions BCG, *Corynebacterium parvum*, levamisole, or autologous vaccines. The results of these substances are still unpredictable, hard to observe, difficult to reproduce, and hence controversial. Yet those who have had long enough experience of the various procedures of immunotherapy are convinced that "something is going on," and that we may not be far from very exciting results. They are also convinced that if it is well handled, immunotherapy is not dangerous, or at any rate that it is less dangerous than any other therapeutic method. In theory, therefore, there is a place for various types of immune stimulation whenever a cancer patient presents a weakness of immunity, whether that weakness antedates the cancer, accompanies it, is caused by it, or is produced by treatment.

But there is an enormous gap between granting that, in theory, immunotherapy has a place in treatment and proposing that it be used systematically. That gap can be closed only by years of clinical and basic research, but it is research that must be done. Recently a prominent lung specialist said confidently, "Show me one single case of bronchial cancer that has been improved by immunotherapy, and I'll begin to believe in it." An imprudent statement. It so happens that if a bronchial cancer were already evident and inoperable, it would never occur to anyone to use immunotherapy alone. The real question is, Does combining immunotherapy with chemotherapy improve the results of the chemotherapy? But who is ever going to provide the answer to that sort of question if not the lung specialists, whose task it is to test hypotheses that might advance the art of curing and not merely to continue treading the beaten paths.

Another problem for the years immediately ahead will be to determine whether, after surgical removal of a tumor, certain types of immunotherapy are likely to improve the long-term results. Cooperative investigations on the subject are being carried out by various international teams, and we will not have too long to wait for their results.

Immunotherapy, then, is the youngest brainchild of medical oncology. It seems to be of sound constitution and promising development. But it still requires close supervision. We cannot and should not
recommend its indiscriminate use. The vast majority of cancer cases
now being treated throughout the world are not receiving it. They may
receive it tomorrow if the work in progress in specialized centers
confirms the hopes raised by preliminary studies.

I do want to report here two striking cases out of dozens that are
good illustrations of the idea that something is going on. A few years
ago, a young woman, the wife of a doctor, consulted us in great alarm.
She had several hundred melanotic tumors on one leg, following a
nevocarcinoma. And her case was indeed highly disturbing, in view of
the number of her tumors and the rapidity of their evolution. She was
very reluctant to undergo chemotherapy, which in any event would
have been of little or no use in such a case. She warily agreed to
intranodular injections of BCG. We began them cautiously, without
daring to use the total dose required. After several weeks, when we had
still injected only a minority of the nodules, she noticed that certain
others that had not been treated were drying up and falling off spontaneously. She had a strong reaction after every injection of BCG and
wanted to stop, but we persuaded her to continue. Then one day we
stopped, simply because she had little by little eliminated the enormous
number of lesions she had had in the beginning. For several years she
has been cured and is leading a normal life. Hers is the only really
convincing case I have been privileged to observe of the effect of local
immunotherapy on distant tumors, but it is enough to prove that the
thing is possible. The rest is a matter of patience, intelligence, and
imagination, qualities that are not lacking in the many teams who treat
these cases.

There is another case that all of us here remember: that of a young
woman suffering from a sarcoma with pulmonary and bone lesions. She
limped, was short of breath, and could not undergo chemotherapy
because the state of her blood was disastrous. On no account would she
agree to be hospitalized, because she was afraid her husband would
leave her. She feared radiation. In short, she was one of those impossible cases in which the medical difficulties are compounded by insurmountable problems of all kinds. Without much faith, but not wanting

to abandon her to her wretched condition, we proposed an immuno-therapy by intravenous injection, which she would come in for while continuing to live at home. In three weeks her condition was trans-formed: the pulmonary lesions diminished by half; she began to wear lipstick again. Unfortunately, she soon abandoned all treatment, in obedience to the wishes of her husband, who did not want her to come regularly to the hospital, and we afterward found out that a few months later the disease flared up with a vengeance. But the documents are there.

It is therefore possible for a "manipulation" of immunity (that is as precise as we can be, given our present level of knowledge) to cause large tumors to regress, at least temporarily, sometimes permanently. To me, these examples confirm the fact that there is hope and that a new weapon has been added to our arsenal.

In a few short years the development of immunotherapy has over-turned a considerable number of dogmas. It seemed established that immunotherapy could be effective only on the minimal residual disease left after an operation. Yet our team has demonstrated that im-munologic procedures, such as plasmapheresis (plasma exchange) or daily intravenous administration of *Corynebacterium parvum,* can bring about regressions in disseminated cancers as well. It also seemed established that chemotherapy and immunotherapy were mutually ex-clusive. Yet we have shown that they complement each other, and this has been extensively confirmed by other teams.

One of the problems that must now be addressed is the fact that, although the mechanisms of immune escape and immune failure are numerous and vary greatly from one patient to another, in most studies the same immunotherapy procedure is prescribed for all. At a sympo-sium held at the M. D. Anderson Tumor Institute in Houston in 1970, I presented a list of mechanisms of immune failure. Most of them relate to the capacity of tumors to paralyze the defenses of the host. These mechanisms are accessible to therapeutic measures, and we already possess the basic technology for treating them. The next step is to undertake controlled clinical trials to check the effectiveness of such treatments. For my part, I am confident that we will see important results in this area in the next few years.

11

❀❀❀

The Combined Strategies

We have now summed up the different methods of treatment. Surgery can remove the original tumor, sometimes completely, sometimes partially, and perhaps an isolated metastasis. Radiotherapy can either sterilize a small tumor, making it unnecessary to remove it, or cause an inoperable tumor to regress for varying periods of time. Chemotherapy, with the limitations we have seen, can reach the disseminated metastases that are almost always present. Immunotherapy can strengthen the organism's ability to defend itself and so help it to tolerate other treatments that are effective but immunosuppressive.

It is difficult to estimate the number of patients who are now being treated by a combination of these different methods, but if I judge by those whom we receive in our unit, and whom we rarely see at the beginning of their illness, it does not exceed 15 percent of the total number of cancer patients. The overwhelming majority of the patients who come to us have never had anything but local treatment, applied to the visible part of the disease: surgery, when it was possible, or radiation, or sometimes, in certain sites, a combination of the two. In a few rare cases of disseminated cancers, the patient will already have had chemotherapy, generally administered in a timid and inadequate manner. And most often, these disseminated cases come to us not because they have been referred by physicians or surgeons but because they have been brought by relatives who, despite the fact that the patient has been advised to abstain from treatment, want to try something.

There are two things I have observed that are symptomatic of the current attitude of the medical profession. One is that the surgeons or radiotherapists who see the patient first almost systematically advise against combining a local treatment with a general treatment designed to combat the invisible residual disease. The other observation is perhaps even more striking: if a patient has both a primary tumor that can be treated and a metastasis, he is rejected by these practitioners. He is either abandoned to his fate or referred to a chemotherapist for what is essentially a semblance of treatment. If the various specialists worked in collaboration, such a patient might have a chance, but local treatments and general treatments are thought of as antagonistic, or at any rate incompatible. It is the law of all or nothing. If the surgeon thinks that he can't triumph over the disease alone, he washes his hands of it. If he thinks—mistakenly, in most cases—that he *can* triumph alone, he refuses the help of general postoperative treatment and advises against it.

These attitudes are based on neither logic nor empiricism. They are purely irrational, and they exert an influence detrimental to patients. They cause doctors to take emotional stands that are sometimes even reflected in the scientific press. Fortunately, however, voices are now being raised in favor of approaches that are more daring and therefore —in a disease where to abstain is to lose the battle—more rational.

In 1967, when I published my first observations on the combination of polychemotherapy and surgery in cases that were supposedly inoperable, I did not succeed in interesting many doctors. Yet I wasn't the only one to whom the idea had occurred. Already many oncologists were combining various modalities of treatment, and observations were being published here and there. Today the quarrels continue—in France, at any rate—among surgeons, radiologists, chemotherapists, and immunotherapists. In the United States, the National Cancer Institute has a special office responsible for elaborating combined therapeutic approaches. The big American cooperative groups, which until now have devoted themselves to chemotherapy alone, are called upon, on pain of having their research funds reduced, to develop treatment protocols using combined approaches in circumstances where chemotherapy, radiation, or surgery was formerly used alone. But here again, these approaches are reserved exclusively for cases that are operated upon, and the greatest timidity still reigns in the treatment of more extensive cases.

If specialists in medical oncology are to elaborate combined strategies, they must first analyze every aspect of each individual case. This preliminary analysis must include the following elements:

- General information about the rate of evolution of the tumor in question, its histological variety, its sensitivity to the different treatments available in the particular context of sex, age, and so forth.
- Evaluation of the patient's immunological condition.
- Assessment of the tumor's local and regional extent, with evaluation of possible disturbances of function.
- Exhaustive assessment of its dissemination at a distance, including various examinations capable of revealing secondary lesions that are otherwise undetectable.
- Evaluation of the rate of growth, on the basis of direct evidence if possible, or if not, from indirect evidence such as the length of time since the symptoms appeared, length of time between intervention and recurrence, and so forth.
- Evaluation of the patient's individual resistance to the disease and to the various treatment procedures that might be applied.
- Weighing of the risks it is appropriate to take in treatment, given the result that can be reasonably hoped for.
- Discussion of these elements with the attending physician, with the family, and whenever possible, with the patient.

This evaluation is decisive. It commits the whole future. It can be carried out, and conclusions can be drawn from it, only by a specialist who is experienced in combined approaches, or else by a group of specialists in different approaches, as in the system organized at Villejuif long since by Professor Pierre Denoix. I don't know precisely how these commissions function at Villejuif. But I tend to think that there is no such thing as a decision made by a committee and that, in the end, final responsibility is always assumed by one person alone. This raises the question of that person's character—which medical school examinations are not designed to evaluate—and the question of his training—which is a difficult problem in a field that is constantly changing. Again I draw attention to the fact that 80 percent of French cancer patients are not cared for in cancer centers, and I am almost sure that this is the case everywhere. And I want to repeat how often my associates and I are distressed to see patients who have been given first one treatment by a surgeon, then another by a radiotherapist, sometimes another by a chemotherapist, all without any coordination. Very often the treatments haven't been applied in the correct order. It depends on chance, or the reflexes of the attending physician, who in any event does not know any oncologists because there are not enough of them, and refers his patients to a general surgeon who has become accustomed to making decisions in an area that is beyond his competence.

The few general oncologists practicing today have been trained on the job and are almost always physicians. Not because physicians are more competent, but because they don't have to master and apply the particular techniques of surgery or radiotherapy, which are very time-consuming and lead to overspecialization. Thus it is more appropriate for the general oncologist to orchestrate combined approaches, and more compatible with his training not to have prejudices against this or that method of treatment. But although I maintain this point of view, I am not going to take up the cudgels in defense of the supremacy of physicians. It would be a great step forward to have among the surgeons and radiotherapists specialists who were able to take the fullest possible advantage of the other treatments. We are beginning to have a few, but we must nurture them carefully, for they are still much in the minority.

Among cancer specialists who claim to belong to the avant-garde, especially in the American cooperative groups, there is still a tendency to take for granted that patients with disseminated cancers can be treated only by various chemotherapies. We know how rare it is that complete remissions are achieved under these circumstances and how precarious even partial regressions are. The treatment plans provide that in case of failure—that is, lack of response, or regrowth of the lesions—another course of chemotherapy will be applied. But every chemotherapist knows that any drug is usually less effective when it is administered as a second treatment than if it had been given from the start. (I have hypothesized that this is the result of a lowering of immunity caused by the preceding treatment.) The patients are not supposed to be given immunotherapy, which, as I have said, many believe—mistakenly, in my opinion—to be ineffective in disseminated lesions. Nor are they given radiation, which supposedly it is too late to apply. Thus, in those cases where a battle is waged, it is already a rear-guard action. We are going to see, however, that even in these cases there is sometimes much that can be done.

We have shown, for example, that immunotherapy and chemotherapy usually have a synergistic effect in disseminated cases—that is, each reinforces the other, producing a very significant prolongation of survival. This concept conflicts with a series of current dogmas, and we ourselves didn't put much faith in it when we began to test it systematically. But all our studies convinced us of its validity, and our work has been confirmed by that of others, the Houston team headed by Evan Hersch in particular. In some severe and extensive forms of lung cancers, certain immunotherapy programs now make it possible for us to obtain complete and prolonged regressions in one out of two cases.

We have one patient who is probably cured today, whom we have been following without treatment for two years after a treatment of three years. He told us that tongues had finally begun to wag in his village. People had admitted to him that at the beginning of his illness (a large and inoperable lung cancer), his family and friends, taking the word of specialists, had abandoned all hope of seeing him live beyond six months. This would have been a perfectly accurate prognosis if no attempt had been made to treat him. But the curious thing is that the cancer specialists in the largest city in his region advised against the treatments his family wanted to try, predicting they would be useless. He had already had a relapse after radiotherapy: he was therefore a condemned man.

Another of my cases comes to mind. This patient too had relapsed after radiotherapy. He too was subjected to three years of immuno-chemotherapy, which his provincial radiologist administered regularly, despite the fact that his willingness to do so made him unpopular with his colleagues. Today this patient too is cured. He is working and has had no treatment for eighteen months. All the tests for cancer cells are negative.

There are other cases as well. We are following patients who were entrusted to us with metastases of cancers of the lung, breast, ovary, and testicle, whom immunochemotherapy has saved from an otherwise fearful prognosis. There may already be cases of this kind who are cured.

One of our patients has impressed me particularly. She was brought to us two and a half years ago with an intestinal obstruction, suffering from a tumor of the cecum that had recurred and metastases in the liver. She was yellow and extremely weak, and the resident who received her in the gastroenterology department where I was to attend her was in favor of abstaining from treatment. The patient wanted to live. We spent three weeks treating her by plasmapheresis, with the help of our machine. She regained strength and improved, to the stupefaction of the team caring for her. Then for a month she was given strong daily immunotherapy, which kept her in an almost constant state of fever. One of her relatives consulted me, very pessimistic, about certain administrative steps. I explained to him what we were trying to do. He gave us permission to continue. The immunotherapy prepared the way for heavy, intermittent chemotherapy, which we then undertook. Today this patient is living at home. She is perfectly fit, suntanned, in good shape. Twice a month she comes for perfusions that make her vomit for three or four hours each time. She has kept her hair. Her tumors have regressed. Nothing in the world would make her abandon her treatment.

Not all our cases are so spectacular. But the duration of comfortable survival is multiplied, on the average, by a factor of three. Which means that for some of the most fortunate cases, it is already multiplied by a factor of eight and some are going to be cured.

The hematologists, who treat cases of Hodgkin's disease and blood sarcomas, already know that adding chemotherapy to radiotherapy significantly prolongs survival in serious cases and produces a marked increase in the percentage of cures.

Most oncologists consider that when the usual cancers are disseminated, radiotherapy, which is only a regional treatment, is no longer indicated. This is a fatal error in reasoning. It is true that one can't irradiate simultaneously—or successively—numerous disseminated metastases without grave danger to the blood. But there are nevertheless many situations in which we can combine these procedures and show that they are complementary. For example, when chemotherapy brings about partial regression of several lesions, there is something more to be done than simply continuing the therapy, hoping for stabilization. Irradiation, in very moderate doses and in narrow beams, of the lesions resistant to chemotherapy can, without major toxicity, secure more important or even complete regressions, and therefore set the illness back. The time gained is precious and can be exploited by other immunochemotherapies.

One day in my office at Lariboisière, I was seeing a patient whose lesions, after partial regression under chemotherapy, were marking time or growing back. My friend Philip Rubin of Rochester was passing through. He advised us to apply a large dose of radiation for a very short time to very limited areas. I had all the trouble in the world finding a radiologist in Paris who would agree to this program, especially as the lesions were supposed to be radioresistant. But it was finally done. For more than two years this patient has been in a state of stable partial remission, under immunochemotherapy.

In other cases, when faced with tumors that are progressing rapidly, we may decide on a different strategy: we will undertake simultaneously —as we have shown it is possible to do—both heavy radiotherapy on the most threatening lesion and a chemotherapy combining two or three drugs that are only very slightly toxic for the bone marrow and hence are compatible with radiation. The addition of an immunotherapy further improves the tolerance of the blood and enables us to exert a degree of pressure on the disease that was impossible a few years ago.

In still other cases, when a discouraged radiotherapist throws up his hands because there are four bone lesions and that means that there will be others and he won't be able to irradiate all of them, we persuade him to make a start. We know that if we then take over with an immunochemotherapy, we may be able to put a stop to the appearance of new metastases, especially if we are dealing with bone lesions from breast cancers, which are very sensitive to chemotherapies and often to hormone therapies that are not toxic.

Four years ago, a young woman was sent to us with multiple lesions, one of which was cranial and threatened the optic nerve, pushing the eye out of its socket. We began medical treatment at once and entreated the radiotherapist—sometimes they have to be entreated!—to irradiate the threatening lesions. He agreed unwillingly, because he was honest, and said to us, "If I irradiate with effective doses everything you ask me to irradiate, I am going to cause bone-marrow aplasia, especially if you administer your poisons besides." But he did agree, and we even persuaded him to administer doses that, while they could not sterilize a local lesion by themselves, would help us considerably as a "reductive" treatment. This young woman is still under treatment today. She may not be cured. But she appears to be cured, lives a normal life, and comes to us every two months from her province. Her radiotherapist, who still can't get over it, says she has been saved by a miracle. It is not a miracle. She is not the only one—far from it. There are many like her, in every country in the world, wherever patients have not been dissuaded from aggressive treatments by timorous therapists.

Another of our patients consulted us in 1971 with metastases in the liver and lungs from a cancer of the breast that had been operated on a few years earlier and not kept under observation. She was given immunochemotherapy and began to improve, but the condition of her liver was still very serious. I had a radiologist irradiate the liver in moderate doses, and this complemented the effects of the medical treatment. The patient went back to work, and one day her husband took her out hunting. On this expedition she met her surgeon, who attacked her vehemently, saying, "If you really had what you say you have, you would be dead or at death's door. Therefore, there is nothing wrong with you. These treatments are unnecessary. You are in the hands of a charlatan." For four years this surgeon was able to rejoice in his opinion. But unfortunately, we were not able to cure our patient completely. The disease was far advanced. In 1975 the hepatic lesions, which had long been contained by constant treatment, resumed their evolution very rapidly.

Another case in which we are combining radiotherapy and immuno-chemotherapy is very instructive for us. It was entrusted to us by a great neurosurgeon of our medical center. The surgical removal of a metasta-sis of a breast cancer had restored a young woman to the appearance of health. A second cerebral metastasis appeared in an inoperable area. The surgeon, consulted again, had the choice of advising abstention, on the basis of virtuous considerations regarding leaving patients to die in peace—advice that would have earned him the esteem of most of his colleagues—or turning her over to us. He opted for an attempt to save her. The patient underwent radiation of the brain, accompanied by a light chemotherapy, which was then followed by a heavy immuno-chemotherapy that lasted a year. We are now in the fourth year. She comes to us once a month for treatment. She is active, lively, in good spirits, no longer has the least paralysis. She insists on stopping all treatment. I dare not give in to her request. I believe she is cured; perhaps I am mistaken. But we have already added two and a half years of active life to her existence.

I have already spoken of "second" surgery in metastases. I want to return to that question in the context of combined treatments. Daring surgeons have always removed single metastases—and their daring generally pays off. If four years after the removal of his original tumor a patient presents a single metastasis, chances are that its removal will again be followed by a long silence and therefore will save his life for another few years. If there are three or four metastases, surgery, even if technically possible, is less tempting, for there is very probably a whole series of metastases that are still undetectable but that will grow and wipe out the benefits expected from the operation. Why not, however, simultaneously institute an immunochemotherapy—which an oncologist will do anyway if he is consulted—and ask the surgeon to remove everything that can reasonably be removed—that is, pre-cisely those voluminous masses that are the least responsive to medical treatment? Obviously, one has to stop somewhere and propose only what is compatible with a quality of survival that is acceptable and comfortable. But it is surprising how much patients who really know what is at stake, or even who merely suspect it, are prepared to accept.

In cases such as those to which I refer, if chemotherapy is followed by recurrences, people will say that it was all useless; if it is not followed by recurrences, they will say that the same result could have been obtained by surgery alone. But we have learned to control our blood pressure when we hear such arguments and to be content with what we know from experience.

Sometimes, of course, we fail. But often we have only failed in part, because between the surgery of the metastases and the new recurrence we have gained for the patient two years of peace, with a resumption of family and social life, renewed hope, and an absence of pain. And sometimes even now we succeed—that is, there is no detectable recurrence three years after the last operation—and in circumstances where such a result would have been improbable, to say the least, in the absence of postoperative treatment.

In certain cases we have even proposed programs including the removal of operable metastases, the irradiation of inoperable metastases, and an immunochemotherapy, and we have "gotten away with it"—that is, we have obtained for two or even three years the appearance of cure, an appearance that in some of our cases is still maintained.

I agree that usually this does not mean a permanent cure such that no further medication is necessary. But I have already pointed out several times that everyone considers an uncertain struggle of this sort perfectly natural when it is a question of cardiac, respiratory, or kidney insufficiencies, or when an organ transplant is involved. I have also pointed out that patients, whether they are told the truth or not, vote for our treatments by submitting to them; besides, they retain the sovereign right to interrupt treatment at any time. I shall add that thanks to these combined strategies in situations where there is dissemination, we are now able to offer more than merely palliative treatments. We think that some of our patients are cured, when otherwise they were unquestionably condemned to death, and what we are learning gives us sound reason to hope that we can regularly increase the percentage of those who are cured. Once again, it's not a question of my personal secrets of success. It is the concerted effort of dozens of teams, in Europe, America, Japan, Australia, South Africa, that makes this regular improvement in results possible. My objective in this book is to make known to those who might be interested that this improvement is real, and that among the cases that are given up for lost, some are no longer completely hopeless and a few are no longer hopeless at all.

No one claims that metastasized cancers are curable today in the same way that localized cancers are. But if we wait to treat them seriously until such time as we have chemotherapies that are sovereign remedies, we are going to lose an incalculable number of years of human lives that could be wrested from death. If we go on mechanically applying the old models of treatment and ways of thinking to these cases, we are letting opportunities for success escape. If even avant-garde groups consider that the only appropriate treatment for such cases is a palliative chemotherapy, clinical research is detoured into paths that have nothing to do with the goals of medicine. By playing on the various possible combinations of treatment and on the particular characteristics of each case presented to us, we are now in a position to pursue the prime objective: individualized therapy so as to do the best we can for each patient.

Let me say once again that there are cases that have gone too far for treatment, cases in which it is the physician's duty to advise abstention. But who is to decide that a case has gone too far? The broader our powers grow, the more crucial this question becomes. As Rabelais says, "Science without conscience is but the ruin of the soul"; and I don't need to be convinced of the profound truth of that remark. But "conscience" without science?

In cases of localized tumors that are inoperable, combined strategies are the answer to a situation in which, so far as the disease is concerned, we have nothing to lose. The surgeon hasn't been able to intervene, or has judged that he wouldn't be able to, or has been unwilling to perform an operation he considered unsatisfactory because it would not completely eradicate the cancer. That being so, we must decide if the other local treatment, radiation, can be useful. At the same time we must bear in mind that when a tumor is large, even if no metastases are yet detectable, there is so strong a probability that they will appear in a short time, that a general treatment should definitely be applied as a matter of course.

There are still very few reliable studies in this area. I shall therefore be obliged to illustrate what could be done by drawing on examples from my own practice.

For lung cancer, the Lung Group of the European Organization for Research on the Treatment of Cancer is conducting a pilot study. All the patients receive radiation, which is certainly beneficial, since even when it's administered alone it can make an inoperable tumor regress or become stabilized. But unlike most radiotherapists, we consider radiation only the first phase of the treatment, and we are studying the effects of applying chemotherapy or immunotherapy, or both, immediately afterward. We are comparing the results of these various combinations to the results of radiation alone. It will be at least another two years before we find out whether we have obtained a significant advantage. Here again, while it is unclear what objections could be made to these studies, we have almost no support from the other Parisian teams. If the lung specialists who advise patients had agreed to collaborate with us, as we constantly suggest, our study would already be complete, and everyone would have an objective means of evaluating combined treatment in such cases.

I should add that it is the same elsewhere. There is a big American organization, the Radiation Therapy Oncology Group, which, under the sponsorship of the National Cancer Institute, recruits as members the cancer radiology centers that are considered the best in the United States. The RTOG did me the great honor of asking me to serve on its Immunology-Immunotherapy Committee. There I was in a particularly good position to confirm the fact that, in medicine at least, conservatism is king. Studies of systematic chemotherapy or immunotherapy following radiation therapy have been delayed for years, for one reason or another, in favor of studies of refinements in radiation technique. My friends Simon Kramer and Philip Rubin, chairman and vice-chairman of the group respectively, are not responsible for this conservatism; it is imposed on them.

Cancers of the ovary are sometimes so widely spread that they can't be surgically removed. In such cases they are either irradiated, if the tumors are no more than three centimeters in diameter, or, if they are larger, subjected to chemotherapy, which is usually based on a single drug. For some years we have been using a different and more aggressive approach, systematically reducing the volume of the tumor by immunochemotherapy. If regression is not complete, radiation is applied, and supported only by immunotherapy for a minimum of a year. This is no panacea. But the results are better than those of the conventional practice and are often excellent. John Lewis, a New York surgeon who specializes in these cases, sent one of his assistants to us for a month to study all our observations in detail and make sure that our conclusions were not dictated by overoptimism. Then he came himself. A fine example of intellectual honesty and openness of mind. Certain surgeons and gynecologists in Paris are aware of our current results because we have treated some of their patients in this way. They have never sent us any others, with the exception of a few Parisian colleagues whom I here thank for their independence of mind and for their confidence in our team.

It seems there is something heretical about our will to fight in cases where many others would resign themselves to the inevitable. Yet the patient who has been under our care the longest already had, when she first came to us, not only a local tumor but also pleural metastases. That was in 1965. Her treatment "cured" her until 1971. Then she had a very unusual relapse, in the form of a pelvic lymph node, which a surgeon removed. Treatment was resumed. This is 1978.

About 15 percent of breast cancers are locally inoperable when they are first seen, because they are already so large or because they are growing so fast. They are usually treated with radiation, and usually successfully. But precisely because they are so large, they have a poor prognosis—that is, a high rate of later dissemination. That is why we decided at Lariboisière to treat these cases simultaneously with radiation and light immunochemotherapy, then to continue with prolonged, more intensive immunochemotherapy. The good results we have obtained, on a short series of cases, are going to be checked by some American investigators. The polychemotherapy we used—one derived from Cooper's studies—happens to be the very one that was used and evaluated for three years by members of the U.S. Eastern Cooperative Oncology Group.

In certain cases of this sort, I did not dare to conclude the program without surgery, for fear of having left in the breast a tumor that was not completely extinguished and might one day start to grow again. It is instructive that recognizable cancer cells were found in none of the cases thus operated upon. Are we going to see a paradoxical situation in which cases that are considered inoperable from the outset are cured without an operation? I wouldn't dare to say so at this point. But in the face of such facts—and I am by no means the only one who has observed them—many of us are wondering about new strategies in breast cancer. Others are shocked that we can so much as wonder. Many physicians have been brought up on the principle that dogmas are sacrosanct. That was perfectly appropriate a century ago, when a medical theory lasted for roughly a generation. Today medical schools should recruit young people who are capable of changing their point of view when necessary. (That is equally true, by the way, for all decision-making positions, in all human activities.)

I could give many more examples, but they aren't necessary to make my point clear. The combined approaches I have mentioned here have already enabled a certain number of cases to move from the category of palliative treatment to the category of curative treatment. Certain patients who couldn't be cured by local treatment alone have now been free of detectable lesions for three years and even five. In other words, combinations of therapies can do for certain cases that are beyond the resources of surgery the same thing that surgery does for more limited cases. Such combinations don't yet give total success—far from it. But the outlook is increasingly encouraging, and for the patients who can be rescued from a hopeless prognosis, we have already won a victory. For others, we have obtained a reprieve that is definitely longer and more comfortable than was previously possible. The patients' families sometimes grow weary, but not the patients, who continue to undergo the treatments with determination. And it is probable that in the years to come, the percentages of success will rise, thanks to better chemo-therapies and also to better immunotherapies. Must we wait until we can cure 100 percent of our patients before we make up our minds to treat them?

So far I have examined situations in which combinations of treat-ment, while they occasionally bring about a cure, basically enable us to prolong survival in inoperable cases where the disease would otherwise prove fatal in the short term. If we now turn to operable cancers, we find situations in which combined therapies make it possible to effect cures on a large scale. I want first to explain how that is possible in theory, and then to analyze supporting examples, many of which have already been published and should be more widely known.

The reader will remember the basic facts about the natural history of cancers. When an operable tumor is detected in a human being, it has passed the thirtieth doubling and contains between one billion and five billion cells. Before reaching this size, it has lost cells, and there has been a constant risk of metastasis. It is therefore likely that there is microscopic dissemination. The visible tumor can—and should—be removed by surgery. But the microtumors will remain, and one day, if they are allowed to develop unchecked, they will again endanger the patient. They are small, generally containing no more than from 10 million to 100 million cells each, sometimes much less. But they exist in a great number of patients: witness the inadequate five-year and ten-year survival rates obtained by surgery alone, rates that are kept down by the development of metastases. These metastases, however, meet almost all the conditions for being eradicated by cytostatic agents: low probability of resistance and a low proportion of dormant cells. Thus it's theoretically possible to achieve excellent results with treatments that are not very toxic. That doesn't mean that in this way we can cure 100 percent of cases. But we have good reason to hope that we will be able to "move the survival curve to the right"—that is, to triple or quadruple the number of survivors at five years, at ten years, and at all the intermediary points. In other words, we think we can achieve an extremely significant advance that will change the outlook for patients who have had surgery. And even if, as we have seen, the drugs now available don't enable us to cure a sufficient number of disseminated cancers, these same drugs should suffice to sterilize the micrometastases, which are much less able to defend themselves, either against cytostatics or against immunotherapy.

Why is it then, since we have already had the drugs for years, that systematic prophylactic postoperative chemotherapy is not more widespread, and that it is even opposed by many surgeons and some physicians? There are two reasons. First, some trials that were conducted more than ten years ago with the techniques of the time, which called for continuous chemotherapy, caused toxic reactions (we now know why) that understandably frightened the surgeons. Rather than make all their patients sick in hopes of a hypothetical result, they preferred to let them lead a normal life after the operation, even though they knew that, depending on the type of case, only one out of two, or one out of four, would still be alive five years later. The second reason is that other trials, which were intended to avoid this overtoxicity, consisted of prescribing postoperative chemotherapies for much too short a time, on the order of one week. As might have been expected, they failed, and the general conclusion was that postoperative chemotherapy was both too toxic and ineffective. That conclusion was wrong on both counts, because it condemned the principle when it should have condemned only the methodology. Readers of science fiction will recognize the precept of Alfred Korzybsky: "In the interest of reason, do not generalize." Years were lost on this account, as we shall see.

But the chemotherapists didn't give up. They learned how to take maximum advantage of their drugs in exchange for acceptable or even zero toxicity. They learned which types of cancers were more likely than others to recur despite a successful operation, and they mounted another assault, treating selected groups of patients in tests conducted at many centers and in many countries, the first results of which are now beginning to be published.

At the same time, other trials were going forward to test the effect on certain tumors of surgery followed by radiation and then prolonged chemotherapy. Still other studies included in addition an immunotherapy designed to stimulate nonspecific immunity, which was sometimes associated with a "vaccination" by irradiated tumor cells from the patient himself or an identical one. I cannot say that these attempts are very popular as yet. Recently a radiotherapist friend of mine, the head of a big radiology department in a hospital, who is hesitant about chemotherapy but has an open mind, said to me, "I'm willing to try with you, but I warn you that my associates think I'm crazy." Let us look at the results, however. This is not a scientific work, and I shall not give bibliographical references for my sources, but it goes without saying that I'm prepared to provide them to any reader who's interested.

I shall not speak at length about Wilms's tumor of the kidney in young children, because I have had no personal experience with it. It is treated, as it should be, by specialists in children's cancer. But the international groups that cooperate in treating these tumors have successively compared the results of surgery alone, of surgery followed by radiation, then of surgery and radiation followed by one or two years of polychemotherapy. They have seen the results improve regularly, from one program to the next. Surgery alone gave a three-year survival rate of 28 percent; surgery followed by radiotherapy gave 44 percent. In 1969, after the first systematic chemotherapies, the rate had reached 54 percent. These results have been further improved since. For localized tumors in children of five or older, the results went from 29 to 73 percent. At present, new combinations of chemotherapy, or immunochemotherapy, are being explored, and the aim is to cure cases that are seen early.

With cancer of the bone, a dread disease, we are witnessing dramatic changes in treatment. Not long ago, after an operation for bone cancer, 90 percent of adolescents died of pulmonary metastases, more than half of which appeared in the first eight months. That is what happened to Pierre Miquel, the son of André, who wrote *Le Fils interrompu* ["The Interrupted Son"]. We fought side by side, but it was too late. The royalties from the book served to equip my laboratory a little better and to perfect some of our weapons. A few years later, things were different for the son of Senator Edward Kennedy, who is at present being treated by my friend Emil Frei in Boston. What had happened in the interim?

I have indicated the results reported by Jaffe and Frei using very strong doses of cytostatics in the treatment of pulmonary metastases from osteosarcomas. These authors reasoned that, in so terrible a disease, they had nothing to lose by applying that same treatment as soon as the operation had taken place, in spite of its toxicity, and applying it for two years, using the "rescue" system of the antidote. At present, in a series in which surgery alone would have given 90 percent relapses, they have only 35 percent! The difference is overwhelming. It justifies all their efforts, all the risks they took, and also all the opprobrium they incurred from conventional physicians. James Holland in New York has had equally fascinating results with another regimen. Of course, combinations of drugs are now being explored, with preliminary results that are even more promising. Donald Morton in Los Angeles and Fudenberg in San Francisco are testing postoperative immunotherapies. A systematic postoperative immunopolychemotherapy for bone cancers will soon be ready. In the last three years, this fearful tumor has entered the group of cancers that are potentially curable. And the same treatments that prevent recurrences are also effective to an extent when the metastases have already made their appearance. To an unprejudiced observer, the argument that chemotherapies should be "reserved" for the time when metastases become clinically detectable is no longer quite so convincing.

With cancers of the breast, we come to what is perhaps the most important point in this whole chapter. Indeed, a veritable revolution in treatment is taking place, and I must describe it in detail.

Some years back, the U.S. National Surgical Adjuvant Breast Project, whose guiding spirit is Bernard Fisher, launched several American groups on a project of postoperative chemotherapy of very short duration—a few days—which was to fail, in that it had practically no influence on survival. Many surgeons loudly rejoiced and declared the very concept of prophylactic chemotherapy to be dead and buried. But Fisher didn't give up. He tried to promote a more effective chemotherapy, of longer duration, better conceived, and yet sufficiently inoffensive to be used on a large scale. At the same time, Paul P. Carbone, chairman of the Eastern Cooperative Oncology Group, was suggesting that we compare the results of treating disseminated breast cancers with a heavy polychemotherapy and treating them with a chemotherapy using a single product administered orally every six weeks. This latter agent was to prove capable of giving objective responses in 25 percent of the cases, which is by no means negligible in the presence of metastases, while the combination of three drugs produced responses in 60 percent of the cases.

From that moment in 1970 on, Fisher, Carbone (who was then associate director of the Division of Cancer Treatment of the National Cancer Institute), and Pierre Band (a Canadian who was chairman of the Breasts Group of the ECOG) conceived the idea of administering this same product, every six weeks for two years, to women who had been operated on for a cancer of the breast with involvement of the lymph nodes. Some fifty American and Canadian units undertook this study in 1972, comparing the results with those of an inert product administered under the same conditions. In January 1975, the publication of the results (which had actually been known to insiders since the previous September) burst like a bombshell: at the end of twenty-four months, the women for whom no chemotherapy had been prescribed —who had simply been kept under observation, as nearly all such patients still are today—were found to have presented many more recurrences than those in the treated group. In the subgroup of patients under fifty years of age, the difference reached a factor of eight! This is an absolutely major breakthrough. The study has proved, for the first time, that postoperative adjunctive chemotherapy is highly effective in the treatment of one of the "common" cancers. But it has proved something else as well. It is now perfectly clear that certain agents that are not very active against disseminated tumors are extremely effective on the postoperative residual disease, on small tumors with more active kinetics. And that is a fact of the utmost importance, albeit one that has gone completely unrecognized: it means that we already possess, and have possessed for a long time, drugs that are capable of eradicating cancers. But we are using them at the wrong time, too late, on giant lesions that are resistant and impermeable, whereas they are active on the smallest tumors, those that remain after surgery and/or radiation have conquered the initial visible lesion.

The history of prophylactic postoperative chemotherapy of breast cancers does not stop there. That would be too simple. Fisher and Carbone were fiercely attacked from all sides, and it is interesting to see how and why.

It happened that on the very day of the first meeting behind closed doors at which the results were analyzed and transmitted to the directors of the National Cancer Institute, an important event was taking place elsewhere in Washington: White House physicians announced the discovery of a breast tumor in the First Lady, Mrs. Betty Ford. Public interest was suddenly focused on the subject of breast cancer, and a few journalists managed to obtain details of the NCI meeting. A heated controversy at once began, with the surgeons and radiologists mounting attacks from different sides.

Some great consulting surgeons of the United States protested loudly that a result obtained at the end of two years was meaningless. Some radiologists, furious because no postoperative radiation had been included in the Fisher and Carbone study, predicted disaster and heaped opprobrium on the National Surgical Adjuvant Breast Project. In October 1974, I invited Fisher and Carbone to come to Paris and present their results before a meeting of distinguished breast-cancer specialists, surgeons, and radiologists. I can testify that they were harried, worn out, and literally shocked by the hostility they had met with at home. Nevertheless, it is they who were right, and I will explain why.

It is absurd to argue that results obtained at the end of two years are meaningless. First, because the time gained is always precious. Second, because the survival curves in almost all studies indicate that a divergence observed at one month or six months tends to grow as time passes, or at least to be maintained. We now know that Fisher and Carbone's results were essentially sustained at the end of three years, especially in the group of premenopausal women, and even more clearly in the group of patients who had less than four lymph nodes involved. Even if the results at ten years do not confirm our present hopes, it is already very important that at two years only 8 percent of the women had relapsed whereas 30 percent had been expected to—as was indeed the case in the untreated group. Is that result too insignificant for the detractors of this study? Will they have to wait ten more years before deigning to take an interest in prophylactic chemotherapy?

Their attitude might be understandable if the result had been obtained at the cost of great toxicity. But that is precisely not the case. The product used, which is administered orally at long intervals, is extremely well tolerated. Critics have raised the specter of possible long-range toxicity. It is not impossible that disturbances might appear in a small percentage of cases. But it is by no means certain, and the advantages of the treatments far outweigh the disadvantages. So on what grounds are they rejected? Let us remember that when patients are operated on for a breast cancer with involvement of the lymph nodes, and given no further treatment, metastases appear in nearly 50 percent at five years, that is, in one case out of two. To persist in abstaining from treatment under these circumstances is incomprehensible, to say the least. So far as the patients themselves are concerned, when I show them Fisher and Carbone's results, they have no hesitation.

As for American radiotherapists, many of them have warned against the absence of postoperative radiation. I repeat that an earlier trial by the Fisher group did not reveal any long-term difference between cases that received radiation and cases that did not. But my personal position is not quite so black and white as Fisher's: to a certain extent, I feel that it does not matter which local treatment is applied. Let the radiotherapists and surgeons agree among themselves which is the most effective and the least harmful—including from the point of view of what will happen later. But then let them agree that the treatment should be completed by a general chemotherapy, the only treatment capable of preventing the development of distant metastases, which are not within the reach of either surgery·or radiation.

The debate continues. By her own report, Mrs. Ford's physicians have subjected her to chemotherapy. Mrs. Nelson Rockefeller, operated on by another team two weeks later, is not receiving any. Let us beware of comparing them, which would be absurd, in view of the disparity between the two cases and the purely anecdotal nature of such a comparison. But one can imagine the atmosphere in the United States, where the statisticians are expecting about 90,000 cases of breast cancer in 1979.

The members of the Fisher group are aware of that prediction. While their first study is going forward, they have undertaken many others as well. In these, the control group, instead of receiving no treatment, is given the treatment that produced such striking results in the first trial.

The group has already completed a second study, comparing treatment by a single cytostatic with treatment by a combination of two. The results have not yet been evaluated. Among other studies now in progress are one comparing two cytostatics with three cytostatics; another comparing the same two drugs with a treatment that also includes an immunotherapy using *Corynebacterium parvum* to stimulate non-specific immunity; and still another evaluating the effects of the anti-estrogen tamoxifene administered after surgery. Taken as a whole, these studies are designed in such a way that in 1980 we should at last have precise, objective, indisputable information as to the best treatment to use after breast surgery in the various subgroups of patients. This is a major undertaking, and one that should be greeted with enthusiasm by all women everywhere, since any woman may one day develop a breast cancer.

I can't end this discussion without mentioning the work of Gianni Bonnadona in Milan. The reader will recall that, in 1970–71, the ECOG compared the results of two treatments for disseminated breast cancers: an oral chemotherapy using a single cytostatic, and a heavy chemotherapy using three drugs. Thereafter, while the Fisher group was exploring the effects of the first of these treatments on women who had had breast surgery, it was suggested to Bonnadona that he study the effects of the second on this same category of patients.

Although less time has elapsed since the completion of Bonnadona's study, it seems that the polychemotherapy he used was more effective for all subgroups of patients on which it was tried than the lighter chemotherapy used by the Fisher group. Now the medical world is waiting for a comparison between Bonnadona's treatment and the various treatments applied in the subsequent studies of the Fisher group mentioned above. That will enable us to determine which is the best treatment and what is the lowest price at which a good result can be obtained. Must we use a treatment as heavy as the one tested by Bonnadona? Or can we, with the same security, restrict ourselves to two drugs or even only one? If we do administer an intensive chemotherapy, will there be more complications in the long run? Should we protect the patients with an immunotherapy? The results of this friendly competition—which is really more of a cooperative effort—will soon give us the answers to these questions.

There is one major problem in connection with breast cancers that can no longer be ignored: the problem of mutilation. Everyone can understand the depth and seriousness of the emotional trauma caused by amputation of a breast. Of course, it is probable that a woman of seventy will be psychologically able to accept a mastectomy without too much distress. But what about a woman of forty or forty-five? Many do not accept it or never get over their heartbreak. For a long time, less mutilating partial operations have been proposed, and since the efforts of Crile in Cleveland, these have their fierce advocates as well as their determined adversaries. What a great step forward it would be if relying on the security provided by chemotherapy, we could promise either surgery that would be conservative from the start or reconstructive plastic surgery after two years! I don't say that that's possible now. I do say that it is the next attempt on the agenda, and that the studies already completed have made it conceivable. But also, since I am writing a personal, polemical book, I shall take the risk of making a prediction. Cancers of the breast will soon be safely treated by partial surgery, or by more extensive surgery followed by plastic reconstruction, supported in either case by complementary drug therapy that is not too burdensome. And then we shall see about those resounding declarations that research on the treatment of cancer is at a standstill.

Postoperative chemotherapy has not yet achieved such brilliant results in other cancers, in part at least because very few trials are going forward and even fewer are near a conclusion. It took the faith and talent of Fisher to start things moving in the National Surgical Adjuvant Breast Project, to give it unity and dynamism. But we must also recognize the importance of the dollars from the National Cancer Institute. The Lung Group of the European Organization for Research on the Treatment of Cancer has been pursuing analogous studies for three years, but the organization gives us only its blessing—no money —and we are not nearly so effective as the NSABP. Yet it is surely in the area of postoperative treatment that progress will be made in the treatment of lung cancer. By two years from now we hope to have gathered enough data to measure clearly the possible benefits of radiation, chemotherapy, or immunotherapy administered after the operation, and of their various combinations.

The group's work is partly financed by the French National Social Security Fund, which at the request of the National Institute of Health and Medical Research (INSERM) has agreed to make a contribution to the study. We gratefully acknowledge this financial assistance, but we need other forms of support as well. For example, we would go faster if more patients were entrusted to us to take part in the study. But my friends at the Center for Thoracic Surgery in Paris, which is run by the Social Security administration, have never sent us a single patient out of the several hundred they operate on every year. They are not organized to do it, they say. There is another center in Paris where they operate on a great many cancers of the lung. The surgeons there are hostile to chemotherapy, after having practiced it themselves a few years ago. It is a little as though I, operating on patients without the least competence in surgery, were to deduce that surgery has not yet been sufficiently perfected. All of which means that only a few thoracic surgery centers in the provinces, and some others in Italy, Spain, Belgium, and Czechoslovakia, are carrying on this study, and that they don't have the necessary support of certain persons whose responsibility it is to allow hypotheses about treatment to be really tested. But the impressions these persons may have about one treatment or another are of no interest to patients or future patients. Human beings are fallible; what counts is facts. To be able to establish that the new treatments we are trying are of no advantage would be useful, because we would then turn our attention to other possibilities. To be unable to establish that they are effective, if indeed they are, would be catastrophic, heartbreaking. And this situation is all the more frustrating because just recently a Japanese study reached conclusions in favor of systematic postoperative chemotherapy in cancers of the lung.

I shall stop this enumeration here. I hope the time is at hand when postoperative treatments will be systematically applied to all cancers that require it. But it will still take some effort to bring that about. In the course of my professional life, I have been surprised to learn that an improvement is not necessarily put into practice automatically, and that it may even arouse the righteous indignation of conservatives. But in the history of new treatments—that is, basically, in the medical history of the last thirty years—truth has always made its way pretty quickly, because it is a question not of academic debates but of the fate of individuals. Patients aren't interested in the personal feelings of doctors who prefer radiotherapy to surgery or vice versa, or in the "impressions" of those who, in defiance of all logic, compare local treatments with general treatments. Patients will turn increasingly to those who have gone beyond quarrels between different schools, to the men and women who have learned and are learning the strategy and tactics of combined treatments.

As soon as there are a sufficient number of such specialists, patients will be referred to them by the general practitioners who, I repeat, are not enemies of progress—quite the contrary. But their eagerness is dampened by the first nonspecialist consultant to whom they send their patient, a consultant who has his own opinions, his own practices, and his own little theory. He has seldom arrived at these legitimately, because how can one presume to form an "opinion" about the treatment of cancer when one doesn't participate in the great international cooperative groups, when one isn't intimately involved in the life, the exchanges and debates of the scientific community that has taken the problem in hand?

This brings us to the delicate and crucial problem of cooperative treatment tests. But before turning to that question, let us conclude this chapter with a few more examples of combined strategies. The first concerns a man of about thirty who, in November 1973, was discovered to have a rapidly developing fibrosarcoma in one leg. Immediately after the removal of the tumor, his doctor sent him to me for what we thought should be a relatively commonplace postoperative chemotherapy. I began it and asked that the site of the tumor be irradiated and also the lungs, at a low dose. (At that time there was a reasonable doubt as to the effectiveness of pulmonary radiation. But when it comes to the treatment of cancer, my motto is: when in doubt, do it.) As soon as the radiation was ended, however, another tumor appeared above the first, this one also evolving very rapidly. I asked that it be irradiated and surgically removed, which was done. A few weeks later there was another recurrence. Everyone became discouraged: the attending physician, the family, the patient (who was aware of the diagnosis), and the surgeon, who blamed me for not having had the leg amputated. I had refused to do that because until we were able to control the tumor medically, there was no point in extensive surgery: another tumor would surely appear above the amputation. We changed the chemotherapy and decided to apply a local immunotherapy, in the hope of destroying the tumor and possibly stimulating a favorable immune reaction. We succeeded. The treatment was continued for several months. A year after the first operation there were no metastases. The last recurrence had been controlled.

I then decided it was time for the amputation and proposed it to the patient. It was performed below the knee by an excellent orthopedist. The general treatment continued. A few weeks later, however, another small tumor appeared on the scar. It was excised, but everyone had begun to lose hope. We changed to still another chemotherapy, of the type developed by Jaffe and Frei for bone tumors. Another few months of struggle and another recurrence near the scar. However, it was small and slow, and thank heaven there was still no sign of metastases at a distance. I asked my friend Morton in Los Angeles for advice. He cabled me proposing an intra-arterial perfusion with a new cytostatic for three days, and a second amputation, this time at mid-thigh. At first the patient refused. He did not want to lose his knee, which had made it possible to fit him with an acceptable artifical limb. I convinced him. I convinced the orthopedist. Morton's plan was carried out and the amputation of the thigh performed in the autumn of 1975, nearly two years after the onset of the disease.

Unfortunately, the patient, who again plunged into active life, broke off contact with us for six months, stopped all treatment, and persuaded himself that he was cured. What a mistake! He came back to see me with a pulmonary metastasis. It is he who is now in Boston, in the hands of the Frei team. Two and a half years of struggle, for an uncertain result. But he is one of the patients who not long ago had a life expectancy of three months, some of whom we are going to cure. He is fighting, with his young wife and two children at his side. I saw him after his last relapse, and he was once again ready for anything. I believe he is grateful to the medical profession for not capitulating. Indeed, it never occurred to the Boston doctors to capitulate: they immediately threw themselves into the battle.

Over the past four years, we have received in my unit three similar cases, seen after many relapses. With one of them, a young boy, we lost the fight, after two years of struggle. The two others, a young woman and a man of fifty, have been free of any visible lesion for three years, and I have dared to stop their treatment. Every time I am to see them again, I feel a weight of anxiety that is not lifted until I have seen the results of all the tests. For years my associates, my nurses, and I have been living in this atmosphere of front-line combat, without letting ourselves be disturbed by the disapproval of physicians who think—and proclaim—that we are "overdoing it." How can we give up trying when we know that the chances of success are increasing all the time?

Combined strategies are also valuable in defensive situations. In 1970 a patient of forty-five was operated on for a tumor of the mediastinum. The surgeon was not able to do what he had hoped. He asked for radiation, which was given but was not enough to eradicate everything that remained. The patient was then referred to me, not by either his surgeon or his radiotherapist but by a friend of his who happens to be a doctor. He received two years of a chemotherapy that some would call hard, but he took the treatment regularly without flinching, every two weeks, and continued to work. He implied that he was aware of the real situation but didn't ask me any direct questions. After two years everything seemed to be going well. I lengthened the time between treatments, then stopped them entirely. Six months later there was a recurrence. Many drugs had already been used and had become inactive. The patient's condition did not allow of another intensive chemotherapy. I instituted an immunotherapy, flying in the face of all the dogmas according to which immunotherapy is ineffective in disseminated cases. This treatment blocked the evolution of the tumors. In a few months it made it possible for us to resume an oral chemotherapy that strengthened our control of the disease.

Since then the lesions have not really diminished, but they are not growing. That has been the position for more than five years, during which our patient has been hospitalized only once, for a period of three weeks. He is not cured in the full sense of the word, but we have transformed an explosive disease into a chronic disease, at the cost of a treatment that has been sometimes hard but acceptable, and in any case accepted. The patient has not shared with me his changing emotions over those five years. Unlike the preceding case, our relations are of the kind that consist of the somewhat lingering look, the discreet half-smile, the short silence. But his courage, his confidence, and his adherence to our successive tactics have brought him to his present position—that is, to an independent existence, without a physical handicap other than the treatment, which is now administered every four weeks, and which he would like very much to be able to stop entirely someday.

The last "story" is to me one of the most moving. A woman, well known in her own country, was brought to us one day by a French doctor who is a friend of hers. Metastases from a breast cancer were causing such pain in her spinal column that she couldn't bear to stand. A few weeks earlier, she had undergone an operation for decompression of the spinal cord and also radiation. She was faint from pain. She knew everything about her condition. I entreated her to remain in Paris for the first part of her treatment, which would include additional radiation because I was not in agreement with the radiation program she'd had, and also a chemotherapy and an immunotherapy. Five weeks later, in good shape morally and physically, she went away, leaving me worried about what was going to happen next. But she pursued the treatment with unbelievable energy. She endured everything. She fought back. A few months later she resumed her activities, which were very much in the public eye, surprised all of her friends who "knew," and told the others, "It was only a cancer metastasized to the bones, and I'm much better now."

A year after her first visit, she announced to me that she was starting life over again with a man to whom she had told everything, and said, "If it is a temporary reprieve, I want to take advantage of it. If it is more than that, all the more reason." She lived for thirty months after our first meeting, and died in Italy from a pulmonary infection. Her doctor at the time felt it was useless to fight again!

Of course these are encouraging examples. There are others that are less encouraging. But already there are these. We need no longer assume automatically that it is impossible to control cancer. Thanks to the combined—and obstinate—use of the weapons that different disciplines have placed at our disposal, the disease need no longer follow a blind and ineluctable course. That is the important thing. It is into that breach that we must pour all the resources of our intelligence, our imagination, and our will. Little by little, the breach is already widening. There will come a day—and I believe it is not far off—when the walls of the fortress will crumble. If, in the meantime, our scientists have discovered the ultimate causes, the intimate mechanisms of cancer, and the absolute weapon against it, so much the better. But whether or not they have been able to do so, we will have proceeded like the engineers we are. We have probably not yet heard the last word about the form and function of the internal-combustion engine, but the automobile industry is not doing too badly.

Part Four

❀❀❀

ATTITUDES TOWARD CANCER

I know of no other area of medicine in which there is so great a gap between the theoretical possibilities of available treatment and daily practice. Medicine is in general a privileged field in which, as soon as a theory is put forward, it is verified in practice, and sometimes it is even practice that dictates theory. That is because we are here to save lives or to relieve suffering, and we are in a hurry. We are concerned with individuals who are in pain or whose lives are threatened. This explains the pragmatic side of the physician, who can't afford the luxury of really being a "scientist," and who judges his decisions by the effectiveness of his treatment. If "it works," everything is all right.

Yet in the field of cancer, where we have less to lose than in many others, we make only the most timid advances. Approaches that groups of specialists have been advocating for years are not even given large-scale trials, and a great number of physicians are perfectly content to go on living without ever really finding out if "it works." Let us try to analyze what is going on, to see how—and maybe why—doctors and the public conspire to maintain this resistance to progress.

12

❀❀❀❀

The Public,
the Patient,
the Truth

A great deal is being written about cancer currently, and I am told that films and television programs on the subject have a wide audience. The specialists are making commendable efforts to convince the public that cancer can be cured—which is true. Yet, on the one hand, the fundamental pessimism of the public remains untouched by these campaigns; on the other, the idea of death, which in our culture is identified with the idea of cancer, has never been more dreaded nor less accepted than it is today.

The demands on the medical profession and the public authorities are not expressed in the name of the people's right to health care but in the name of the people's right to health; the death of a close relative is perceived as a failure or an injustice, not as an inescapable event. In short, people are no longer willing to die. Or even to cross swords with death. The driver on a holiday weekend, the mountain climber, and the criminal persuade themselves that death is for other people—hence their sense of security. The cancer patient, however, is persuaded that he is doomed—hence the heavy silence and the extreme difficulty of finding a correct solution to the problem of whether to tell him the truth.

Early in my career I had an experience that I have never forgotten.

At the end of my residency, having successfully defended my thesis, I had gone into private practice while waiting to take the examinations for a full-time affiliation with a hospital. It was the first time after eleven years of study that I was seeing patients in my own office, that I had leisure to deal with any problems that were not strictly technical, and that I became aware of the need for a deeper relationship between doctor and patient.

For the most part, I was seeing patients with pulmonary diseases, and several times I had occasion to reassure men who mistakenly believed they had a lung cancer. I was struck by two things: first, that a profound breakdown of the personality accompanied their fears, occurring suddenly even in men who were very self-possessed and sure of themselves, men who held important positions; and second, that as soon as they were reassured, they immediately forgot their terror, regained their good spirits, and once more radiated confidence. I was thirty, and I had more illusions then than I have today. I conceived the mad design of making myself useful to these men over and above what they were asking of me: I would try to help them mature in these crisis situations so that another time they wouldn't let themselves be caught off balance.

I remember that on several occasions, highly pleased with myself, I made the following sort of speech: "I am delighted to be able to reassure you completely. You do not have cancer. But when you thought for a moment that you did, you collapsed. And now with one stroke of the pen you write off the possibility that one day you might again be in danger. Yet you know that you and I both belong to a mortal species. Someday, alas, for one reason or another, your fears will be justified. Will you again collapse, or will you take advantage of the present ordeal to meditate, to free yourself gradually from this fear, and when the day comes, to confront your destiny calmly?"

It took no more than a few embarrassed remarks by mutual acquaintances, all to the same effect, to make it clear to me that my statements verged on the obscene. All I was asked to do was to reinstill confidence, a sense of comfort, and blissful ignorance. Not only was it not my business to "preach"—a proposition to which I humbly agree—but, I was told, I had revealed a sadistic streak that was really disturbing in a physician.

So I resolved to hold my peace, realizing that in this particular culture my basic mission was to deny death, never to speak of it even as a remote possibility, but on the contrary to incarnate the figure capable of exorcising it.

In the light of this sort of experience, the vehement statements of persons in good health who demand that those who are going to die be told the truth now leave me somewhat cold. Not that I underestimate the importance of the problem of telling the truth, or that I think I have resolved it. I only consider that there is more than one dimension to it, and that my profession requires that I take each of them into account.

Freud says somewhere that the subconscious always believes itself to be immortal. That is probably true, except for the subconscious of cancer patients. For many complex reasons, Western man has a deep-seated conviction that cancer is the sickness that can never be cured. He sees it as the work of the devil, the malady from which there is no reprieve, and he deeply resents the idea that if he is stricken with cancer, he has truly lost the immortality that was otherwise his portion.

It is not my purpose here to interpret this phenomenon, nor am I competent to do so, but clearly it exists. For how else are we to explain the striking difference in the way people behave when they are faced with cancer and when they have, for example, a serious cardiovascular disease? Certain cardiovascular diseases are fatal, certain cancers can be cured. But the two illnesses are not experienced in the same way by the collective consciousness or by individuals. Doubtless it will take a very long time for that to change, and one can easily imagine that a sudden, spectacular advance would be much more effective in bringing the change about than the slow progress we have been making during the last few years. A magic pill that would immediately enable us to shout "Cancer has been conquered!" would be a powerful charm, capable of making men invulnerable again. But when we say, "In such and such a form of cancer we have increased the number of cures by 20 percent in two years," people think vaguely either that that is not completely true, or that the improvement may be valid for others but not for themselves. Hence the tendency to seek out a charlatan who, using "unofficial" methods, can put himself on the plane of magic and, with the rites of exorcism, reestablish "order." Hence also the great complexity of the question of whether to tell patients the truth.

To say to a patient "You have a cancer" is to say much more than "You have a serious disease"—even, sometimes, more than "You have a disease that may be fatal." In our cultural context—at least on this side of the Atlantic—to say that is to rob the patient of his soul, to consign him to hell, to inflict on him the ultimate trauma. Doctors have always felt this, and up until now the vast majority of them have refused to tell the naked truth. As everyone knows, they are subject to all sorts of pressures. They are even accused of robbing their patients of their deaths. However, I must say—without lessening the reservation I shall express afterward—that the position of French doctors, for example, is collectively much more responsible, much more courageous, than that of American doctors, who, for reasons that are not always pure, tell their patients the "truth" straight out and leave them to digest the news.

It is true that almost all doctors on the other side of the Atlantic live under the threat of being sued for malpractice—which, by the way, is a most distressing and frightening phenomenon of civilization. They must therefore justify every therapeutic measure, discuss their choice, secure the patient's consent. And that means there must be almost total truth. The patient is told not only that he has a cancer but that he has hepatic metastases that will probably evolve in such and such a way. My colleagues have explained to me a hundred times over that their relations with their patients, and the patients' relations with their families, were the better for it, and that they would reveal the truth even if they were not obliged to do so. But I remain skeptical. It is true that Americans are more willing to accept the possibility of death than we French are. Nevertheless, in the United States as in France, I have seen cases of helpless anguish.

We must also add to this debate another aspect that's often forgotten: there are an infinite number of patients who, without ever admitting it to others or to themselves, "know." Something in them knows. Yet for a variety of reasons they don't seek to clarify the situation. They don't speak of it to their family. They don't ask their doctor about it. There is, after all, in reply to the advocates of truth at any price, one fact that must be emphasized: the patient very seldom asks for the truth. He undergoes all sorts of treatments, sees his condition fluctuate, is surrounded by menacing problems, and asks nothing. Often he even adopts a complex strategy, proposing explanations and diagnoses first, so that the doctor won't be tempted to supply his own. Is the doctor supposed to break down this resistance and, in the name of the intellectual constructs of persons who are not suffering, to destroy the defenses of those who are? What is the meaning of these defenses? That the patient has a doubt, a doubt he can encapsulate and repress if given the chance, and that he desperately wants to repress. In such a situation, with such a defense mechanism at work, I have never felt I had the right to tell the truth, and I am prepared to defend that position against the criticisms of my contemporaries.

The problem, however, is more complicated than that. There are patients who insist that they want to know the truth. These patients can be divided into two groups: those who really mean it—for all sorts of reasons, religious, philosophical, material—and those who want only to be convinced that they don't have cancer. The latter can neither live with their doubt nor repress it. But they are not interested in the truth. They are seeking an assurance without which life is unbearable to them —even if their cancer is curable. Here again, I hold that even if we were able to identify accurately the members of this second category, we should not tell them the real diagnosis. They are not turning to us as to a computer. The doctor's choice is between truth and charity. And to choose in favor of charity is to render a service far above the kind for which the Social Security Administration can set a fee. Besides, a mistake can be very costly: often it means an incurable depression, which may be more serious than the cancer itself; sometimes it even means a suicide. Hence the natural tendency of doctors in our Latin civilizations to err on the side of falsehood, out of concern for the patients' interests.

But there are also those patients who really do want to know, who want the truth to be spoken in the plainest words, and who accommodate to it, reorganize their relations with themselves and with others on this new basis, and perhaps really do have an important, authentic experience of which neither a doctor nor anyone else has the right to deprive them. Each of us would like to be one of those. It is the very heavy task of the doctor to identify them, to make as few mistakes as possible, in one direction or the other. The knowledge that enables one to give the right answer wherever the question is asked—in the privacy of the office or in front of students, without warning—is not to be found in textbooks. Nor is it to be found in psychiatric journals or magazine columns. It is acquired, more or less successfully, over the course of professional life.

At this point, two further questions must be introduced. First, what is truth? Second, what effect do current technical advances have on the debate as a whole?

One could discourse at length about the content of the word "truth." It happens that the question that is usually asked is not "What is the percentage of recurrences or of metastases after one year, two years, five years?" or "What is the prognosis, given the fact that I have an isolated hepatic metastasis two centimeters in diameter?" Usually the question is "Is it cancer or not? If so, I'm not interested in anything else you may tell me about it. I know that it's all over for me."

This is, alas, a position that is dramatically wrong but that reflects a complex cultural situation beyond the doctor's control, as it is beyond the philosopher's. If the question were posed on an objective level, however, one can see how difficult it would be to give a truthful answer. Because how, in the infinite diversity of clinical situations, can we make a sure prognosis? And how can we temper that prognosis by a calculation of the effect of one or several treatments before we have tried them, before we know how the disease will react, whether the organism will tolerate the treatment, and so forth? There are a few rare patients who question me on that level. Then all I can do is give them the statistics available and tell them why in their case I think we can do better, how far we can hope to go, always leaving a margin of hope that, fortunately, owes less and less to charity and more and more to advances in treatment.

It just so happens—this is the second point—that advances in treatment enter increasingly into the problem of the truth, making it less metaphysical and more technical. An example is the situation in which a treatment that is effective is nevertheless hard for the patient to bear, and he considers giving it up because he doesn't know what is really at stake in the battle he is waging. When it gets to the point where the patient actually wants to stop, must we let him do so, knowing that, out of ignorance, he may be committing delayed suicide? Must we break down the psychological resistance he has organized around the disease and reveal to him the real nature of the struggle taking place? I have no unequivocal answer. It depends on the treatment's chances of success, on the known percentage of cures or the anticipated length of remission, on the psychological structure of the patient and his family, on the nature of the ties that have been formed between him and the medical team. Suffice it to say that it is becoming increasingly difficult for the specialist to keep silent in such a situation. I hope that there will be less and less need for him to do so as our powers increase.

Another situation is even more delicate. A surgeon who has his own reasons to be against any postoperative adjunctive chemotherapy has removed a cancer of the stomach (five-year survival rate: 10 percent), and has advised the patient to rest in the country and not take any treatment, which would be completely unnecessary, since the surgeon has cured him of his ulcer. As is often the case, the attending physician refers this patient to us for a second opinion, but unfortunately after the operation, so that we have no opportunity to let the patient know in advance that postoperative treatment is indicated.

We study his file. Although the tests going forward in various parts of the world are not yet finished, we think, on the basis of the preliminary results and by analogy with Fisher and Carbone's study of the breast, that eighteen months to two years of postoperative chemotherapy would considerably increase his chances of recovery. We therefore tell him that, contrary to his surgeon's advice, we would prefer to prescribe and supervise a course of treatment for him. He refuses and is angry that there is disagreement between two consultants. What should we do? Give in, sick at heart? Or explain what is at stake, with all the serious disadvantages described above? Everything would have been so simple if the surgeon had been content to say, "I have taken out your stomach; it is for the doctors to decide if complementary medical treatment is required." It would also have been simple if we ourselves had been able to refer the patient to the surgeon after telling him the course of treatment we had in mind. With increasing frequency I decide to "tell the truth" in order to give the patient the best possible chance, trying at the same time to de-dramatize the situation as much as I can. There are doubtless patients today who are not receiving the treatment to which the level of our knowledge entitles them, because the dialogue got off to a bad start and because some of the doctors consulted insist that there should be no treatment. Only our advances will enable us to convince the reluctant physicians and also sometimes to reveal directly to the patient the truth that has been hidden from him for mixed reasons.

I have tried in this discussion to indicate the complexity of the present situation rather than to make a judgment about it. Here are a few examples.

A young woman comes to live in Paris after undergoing surgery in Montpellier for the removal of a tumor of the endocrine pancreas that showed signs of developing in a disturbing way. She has been placed on chemotherapy by the doctor at the cancer center who refers her to me. We take over from him without the patient's asking any questions. After eight months of treatment, everything is in order, which is very encouraging, and our patient begins to grow weary of the weekly perfusions. She wants to stop coming for treatment and confides her intentions to my head nurse. My head nurse—to whom I here pay tribute for, among other things, the kind of relationship she is able to build with so many patients—advises her to have a long conversation with me first. In the course of this conversation, the patient asks me what she really has. I tell her, in detail, and reveal to her that partly because of a certain drug we receive from the United States, and other products associated with it, she belongs to the first group of patients in Europe whom we hope to cure, but at the cost of a treatment that is still very prolonged and difficult (she vomits for several hours at a time, once a week, despite the antiemetics). Today we have passed the two-and-a-half-year mark; she is doing very well, takes the treatment regularly, and is going to recover. But she had to admit to my head nurse, after our conversation, that she had been literally shocked by my words, that she had no suspicion of the real diagnosis, even though she had been operated on in a cancer hospital, and that she had been on the point of abandoning the whole treatment. Today, when I tell her that we are going to stop the treatment at the end of three years, she asks me to continue for another six months.

The second example I want to give is one that surprised all my associates. Another young woman was referred to me by her surgeon after the partial removal of an invasive tumor of a rare type, and on her first visit she asked me very resolutely to give her the diagnosis, explaining that she would not submit to treatment unless she was convinced that I was not hiding the truth from her. She was obviously a stable, sensible person. She convinced me. I explained to her, in the presence of my associates and our nurses, what had happened and why she should be treated. She listened without flinching, thanked me, agreed to our program, and for three months came regularly for treatment. Then there was an obvious recurrence of the disease. The treatment had been ineffectual. We had to change it at once, add radiation, and adjust the frequency of the treatment sessions. I explained all this to the young woman at length, minimizing the new problems and regretting that I had let myself be so candid the first time. But the answer she made before my astonished assistants was, "I don't care about all that, Doctor, and I'll do what you want. Ever since you explained to me that I don't have cancer, I am ready for anything."

Here is still another case. An English Canadian, tall, athletic, controlled, and masterful, the head of a company, came to me from the Mayo Clinic and said, "Doctor, my surgeon told me that I would send him a card at Easter, but not at Christmas, because I'll be dead. Can you give me more time?" His voice was a little tense, but he gave no sign of anxiety. I was impressed by this adult behavior, which is rare. I studied the whole file. When I was through, I told him that in my opinion his surgeon had been pessimistic, and that such and such a strategy, based on the fact that his tumor obviously had a slow rate of growth, should give us at least eighteen months and, who knows, perhaps much longer. He discussed all my arguments and had me explain my reasons for each proposal. When I finished, he burst into tears.

Let us move on to those patients whom I call "autonomous." Recently one of them, replying to a journalist who was interviewing him in our unit about the struggle we were waging, said, "There is no such thing as a short period of survival." But another, an American in New York, to whom a second operation had been suggested, said to me, "Doctor, think your answer over carefully. I am willing to be operated on again to gain a year or more. But three or four months don't interest me. I have made my peace with myself. I don't need them." Each of these men stated what was true for him, and in both cases the physician had to stand aside, forget his own philosophy, prejudices, and ideals, and simply serve the patient. Have I, by these examples, convinced at least a few readers of the complexity of the problem? I have no cut-and-dried solution to offer. I believe there is none, and that any solution that lumps all cases together is necessarily false or dangerous. We must leave it to the physician to find the best individual solution in each case, on the basis of his experience, his psychological insight, and the evolution of the medical situation. I sometimes wish I could live in a world in which these relations would be played out between adults, persons who knew the meaning of life and of death and who, while not immune to fear, were not the prisoners of fear.

I have the greatest admiration for the oncologists who work with children and the leukemia specialists, because I know what they go through and that they lose a portion of their substance with each little patient. And I have no personal experience of telling the truth to children. Our patients, who are adult in years, are not always adult in behavior. But who can blame them? Emotional regression due to illness is something that does occur, and which of us can safely assume it will never happen to him? That is why we must be careful of the virtuous demands made by persons in good health. However, if we recognize infantile regression in certain patients, there is a great temptation for us to play the father. Is that really justified? It is easy for the doctor to exceed his role and to manipulate the relationship of dependency in such a way as to impose his philosophy of life on the situation. And the danger is even greater if the doctor is unconsciously busy exorcising his own demons through that relationship. I no longer believe it is possible to practice medicine without basing it on a truly ascetic, daily, profound personal questioning of one's ultimate purpose, taking into account as many facts as possible in all their diversity and not letting oneself be influenced by the dispensers of free advice or the ideologists, for whom everything is simple and who find an answer for everything in their little books.

It is strikingly clear to me that to introduce medical students to inner problems of this sort would be infinitely more useful and responsible than to recruit them on the basis of their knowledge of mathematics. But that is another story.

•   •   •

The attitude of the patient's family is often a problem. Of course we have received any number of letters from husbands and wives of patients, from children and parents, thanking us for the efforts we have made, the results we have obtained, the personal relations that have been established. Often, too, we are thanked for having been able to hide the truth from the patient to the very end. And I frequently have the impression that we have really waged a common struggle, that in our cooperation with the family everything has been dealt with on a rational plane.

But it is not always so. We occasionally witness rejections that are terrible in their cruelty. The patient has been hospitalized for one reason or another. He is better, he is going to leave. A thousand reasons why he should not come home are then advanced by the family, even when he has been eagerly looking forward to the return. We may even be told, as we were once by a young woman, "You can keep him; I have a horror of that disease." And curiously, it is those same persons who send us hostile letters, blaming us for not having been able to effect a cure or for having been lacking in humanity.

Then there are the spouses who don't want to hear the truth. They are in exactly the same psychological situation as the patient. They can't bear it. They come to all the appointments but enter a few seconds after the patient and leave a few seconds before, so as to be certain to avoid a confrontation with the doctor. We suffer from this situation, which often prevents us from finding out enough about the patient to develop a reasonable strategy or to prevent the appearance of psychological, occupational, or administrative problems. And some-times, playing the game to the end, husbands who have never asked us anything take us violently to task when there is a turn for the worse, as if it were the result of an error on our part.

In certain cases, each of the two parties thinks, mistakenly, that the other does not know the truth, or pretends to think so in order not to have to talk about it. In another instance, a wife begs us not to give radiotherapy, even when it might be very valuable, because that would be to admit the truth. In equivalent clinical situations, some relatives ask us to "go all the way," others to stop all treatment. What are we to do when the father begs us to hide the all-too-certain prognosis, and the young wife insists that we tell the "whole" truth?

Doctors who have a member of their family under our care are no different from the others. Sometimes they are more irrational. Some of them, when it is a question of their own wives, are able to overcome their aversion for the disease they fear and bring the patient to our treatment sessions. Gradually, when the situation justifies it, they regain confidence, are surprised at the extent of the improvement, and thank us warmly. But they will never send us the patients they discover in the course of their own practice. Do they go on telling families, "There is nothing that can be done"? I have been asking myself that question for years.

To whom do families turn when they hear that? The question is not hard to answer. It is said that in France there are more charlatans than there are doctors. One might think that, with advances in medicine, they will gradually disappear, but I predict that they will do nothing of the sort. Medical advances increase the tendency of the ill to seek out quacks. When people can't accuse medicine of failing to cure, they blame it for curing by unnatural means. As if the human intelligence were not a part of nature.

And of course it is in the field of cancer that this sort of activity flourishes. As I have said, there is great demand for it, because cancer, which is thought of as a curse, must be conquered by means other than those of science. What is needed is an aura either of secret "powers" and hidden means, or at the very least, of knowledge persecuted by society. Recourse to the irrational is expensive, is not reimbursed by Social Security, and is not tax-deductible. None of that would matter if it were effective. Unfortunately, it is only a ghastly farce.

Let us try to sketch a portrait of the charlatan. He generally has testimonials from well-known respectable personages, but they always belong to the world of law or literature or entertainment, never the world of medicine. He presents himself as a victim of "official" medicine, which would rather see its patients die than admit itself defeated by a "parallel" medicine. He is also the object of a veritable conspiracy on the part of those who mean to preserve their privileges and maintain the status quo, those who fear the truth, and so forth. The remedy he proposes is always based on the observation and utilization of an elementary phenomenon that has escaped the notice of his official colleagues, men less gifted than himself. Preferably an imbalance of some sort—every charlatan has his own—psychological, sexual, or having to do with relations between acid and base, oxygen and carbon dioxide, mineral salts, trace elements, and so forth. One of them has written that it is all right to eat meat providing it comes from an animal that can be caught by hand, or vegetables providing they grow within a radius of fifty kilometers of one's birthplace. Otherwise, beware of cancer. Others effect their cures by reversing the "magnetic flow." But some, like the famous Naessens, have identified the cancer microbe in the blood and have simply manufactured the corresponding serum. Still others extract from human urine or from the organs of various animals anticancer substances that have slipped through the nets of the researchers and that correct the above-mentioned imbalances.

All these remedies (of course there are hundreds more) have one characteristic in common. For various reasons, they have never been subjected to the different tests that are required either by law or by organized research teams. Their chemical structure is partly or completely unknown, and their effects on the normal physiology of various organs and on cancer tissue are either never mentioned or classed in the most unlikely categories. What is more, the clinical observations are unbelievably flimsy, glaringly incomplete, or nonexistent. The presence of cancer, or its recurrence, is never proved, documents are unavailable and are replaced by testimonials from patients, and there is never any indication of the rate of response or its distribution by type of tumor. A precaution that is often unnecessary anyway, since these remedies bring about a cure in almost every case. There was a celebrated Bavarian clinic where out of 570 cases, 93 percent were reported cured. A commission of the Medical Research Council of Great Britain had to go there in order to discover the total and absolute worthlessness of the treatment. A very costly treatment, because the charlatan has his expenses, he prepares his own remedy by small-scale methods.

Against the avalanche of arguments put forward in defense of the charlatans, I will only say:

- No one should imagine that there is any sort of complicity among doctors. The ways of the profession are merciless. Cancer specialists don't treat each other gently. Every "success" is immediately verified by numbers of teams around the world who have no hesitation about publishing counterarticles indicating that the results set forth by so-and-so were not reproduced. Medical journals reject articles that are written obscurely or that don't contain enough details to enable another researcher to reproduce the original work, down to the smallest technical manipulations.

- Because the rules are so strict, when the medical community does certify the results of a treatment, one can be certain that those results are real. We are still waiting in vain for the charlatans to send to serious medical journals documented articles written in such a way that anyone could check their assertions.

- Practicing physicians realized long ago that they wouldn't get a Nobel Prize and that, in fact, they didn't deserve one. Nobel Prizes are awarded to those who make great fundamental discoveries, like François Jacob, André Lwoff and Jacques Monod, or Renato Dulbecco, Howard Temin, and David Baltimore, and not to those who improve the current level of results by applied research. I hope I will be believed, therefore, when I say that we would not feel frustrated or jealous of the "competition" if the miraculous cancer serum were discovered by a brilliant researcher working alone in some remote mountain village. I even hope to persuade the reader—because it is true—that we would be happy about it. Because it is our business to treat the sick and to cure them if possible, and because we would like very much to see cancer conquered once and for all before we quit the stage. And also because we know that our families, or we ourselves, may be stricken tomorrow, and we would be glad to be able to avail ourselves of the serum in question.

- Unfortunately, we are convinced we must give up hoping for the great discoveries that come out of remote mountain villages, discoveries that spring full-blown from the brow of some superior thinker who doesn't have at his disposal the tools of a modern medical center. If those days ever existed, they are gone forever. Everything that could be seen without the aid of an electron microscope has already been seen. All the correlations that could be made without the aid of many teams, communicating with each other and equipped for extensive data-processing, have already been made. Our knowledge—and therefore our power—is expanding faster than ever before, but that is because of huge investments in manpower, hence in training, and in increasingly elaborate technical equipment. And despite all that, it is still necessary to conduct tests, success in the field being the ultimate touchstone, and it is still true that the literature of cancer contains an overwhelming proportion of negative reports—that is, of unsuccessful trials honestly presented by their authors.

Once again, I don't think the considerations set forth above can in any way diminish the vogue of the charlatan, but I do want to say that in view of our struggles, our disappointments, our suffering in certain situations, and above all, of course, the suffering of our patients and their families, I consider the attitude of the charlatans and their defenders to be indecent.

Yet I am against the concept of orthodoxy in scientific matters. Whether it be the imposition of an official theory of the regime, as in totalitarian countries—witness the famous Lysenko affair in the U.S.S.R.—or the attempt by certain powerful persons in our liberal societies to terrorize the scientific community by financially stifling those researchers who don't fall into line with them. But that is another problem. The struggle against ideological despotism in the sciences is the business of the scientists, of those who submit their hypotheses and results to strict verification by experience. In such a debate, the charlatans are disqualified, along with those who defend them.

13

✿✿✿✿

Doctors and Cancer

It is not enough to examine the public reaction to the phenomenon of cancer. We must also ask why doctors themselves more or less consciously resist the application or trial of treatments developed by a few specialists. And why they resist with such acrimony and passion.

People are always telling me that some doctor with whom I've never had any relations, either professional or social, and who has probably never read a line I have published, has spoken ill of me, accused me of relentlessly treating hopeless cases, of being sadistic, and so forth. I assume that I'm not the only one whose crimes are thus denounced. No doubt similar accusations are made against all the members of that small group of French medical oncologists who, for reasons I have explained, stand fast and fight for the patients entrusted to them. We must try to understand the behavior of our critics not only on a rational level but on a deeper level as well. The very vehemence with which they reject our attempts at treatment is proof that such an inquiry is necessary.

A few years ago a scientist who is not in the field of medicine came to talk to me about his wife, who had hepatic and pulmonary metastases from a cancer of the breast that had been operated on a few years before. Having connections with scientific circles in the United States, he had asked the advice of one of his colleagues at the Rand Corporation, who had suggested that he place his wife in my hands. With this in mind, he had gone back to see the surgeon who had performed the operation—a man I don't know—and had received the following answer, which he reported to me: "There is nothing to be done. If you show your wife to Professor Israël, I won't see her again and I won't see you again!" Unfortunately, the surgeon's pessimism in this case was justified. We tried the impossible, without success, and I suppose the surgeon felt the legitimate satisfaction of a man whose conscience is clear. On another occasion not long ago, friends confided to me that in the course of a dinner, a physician of their acquaintance had accused me of applying inhuman treatments, of being in league with "the Americans," and many other sins.

Not everyone reacts this way. An increasing number of doctors call upon us for members of their own families, and a growing number of physicians and surgeons invite us, Alain Depierre and me, to report on our results, and also refer their patients to us. But there is still a very strong contingent of passionate opponents who, curiously enough, are not necessarily the oldest, and who are to be found as often among surgeons and radiologists in cancer centers as among general practitioners. Their basic argument is that the treatments we have to offer, especially the chemotherapies, do more harm than good and impair the quality of survival, either prolonging it in pain and torment or not prolonging it at all. The fact is that long-term chemotherapies using weak doses, like those that are administered to prevent recurrences of breast cancers, are not harmful or toxic. They may induce a state of fatigue, but they don't disrupt the patient's family life or working life. Those of our patients who are undergoing prophylactic chemotherapy continue to work regularly. The only argument, therefore, that can be made against this kind of chemotherapy following surgery or radiation is that while it isn't harmful at present, it may be harmful in the future. That argument can't be taken seriously when we compare the very slight future risks of treatment with the risks entailed in allowing recurrences to appear without trying to stop them.

Opponents of postoperative treatments often pretend to believe that such treatments have side effects identical to those of the palliative treatments I shall speak of in a moment. Even in cases where it is only a question of immunotherapy, the effects of which are entirely different from those of the cytostatics, they oppose the treatment on one pretext or another. An American surgeon (the French are not the only ones who resist) told me not long ago that he didn't feel he had the right to inflict BCG scarifications on patients who'd had lung surgery, because they can leave unsightly scars on the arms. This is the same man who two years ago, feeding data on thousands of cases into a computer, established that patients who had had lung surgery and presented positive lymph nodes had a five-year survival rate of only 18 percent.

I have already described how violently Fisher and Carbone were criticized in the United States. The debate goes on in the pages of the *New England Journal of Medicine*, and certain American oncologists don't hesitate to join in the attack. The argument they use is either foolish or dishonest: we must wait ten years, they say, before we can know if the proposed prophylactic treatment of recurrences is really effective. I call that dishonest because in view of the fact that they refuse to let their patients take part in these trials, how can they expect ever to have an answer? I also call it dishonest because, as I said before, they should at least give credit to the treatment for what it has already accomplished: at the end of three years there were about eight times fewer recurrences! They are so blinded by passion that they refuse to recognize this difference, which is already highly significant if it is measured in terms of suffering and dread.

Let us take up the most thorny problem, the problem of palliative chemotherapies for disseminated tumors. Only ten years ago these treatments were still poorly classified, not very active, and unnecessarily toxic. At that time there was good reason to hesitate between abstaining from treatment and applying a treatment of doubtful effectiveness. In addition to causing fatigue and loss of weight, the chemotherapies sometimes resulted in almost constant vomiting, or in severe infections induced by the lowering of immunity.

It must be admitted that for certain drugs, vomiting is still a major obstacle today, one that is overcome with greater or less success by antiemetics. The vomiting varies: sometimes, as the result of a real process of conditioning, it appears even before the injection; in other cases it is completely absent. The doctor who finds a way to control it will perform an immense service. But we must remember that in the vast majority of cases, the vomiting occurs only during a few hours after the treatment. If the treatment is administered correctly—that is, intermittently—the vomiting is rare. In many cases in which we prescribe a strong chemotherapy every four weeks, the patient vomits one afternoon a month. It is disagreeable, but we warn him about it ahead of time, and we ask him to put up with it as the price of the security the treatment confers. What do you think happens then? The patient agrees to the treatment. Besides, who would dream of forcing him? Ninety-five out of a hundred of our patients live at home and come to our treatment sessions. They could easily avoid them, assuming that this was the only way of escaping from a therapy that impaired their health. But they come regularly, and in increasing numbers, as the administrative statistics of our unit show. Every year there are two or three cases in which we have to break off treatment on account of the vomiting. Sometimes all we have to do is change drugs or suspend treatment for three weeks or have a serious talk with the patient, in order for the vomiting to diminish or to be accepted.

As for the other drawbacks of chemotherapy, they have largely disappeared, at least in units where the therapy is given by qualified physicians. Intermittent treatments that are closely monitored and administered by someone who knows what he is doing rarely cause infections, except in cases of hematological disease. (In such cases it may be necessary to cause a bone-marrow deficiency if the treatment is to be successful, and sterile chambers are required.) Here again, the proof is that our patients live at home, coming once a week for a blood count and a general check-up and receiving their treatments at the prescribed intervals.

One thing more: as I have said, the study of hundreds of measurable cases has shown that when a treatment is going to be effective, its results can be seen very soon. In from three to five weeks, the tumor either regresses or stops growing. This means that we have objective criteria that enable us to tell very quickly when a particular polychemotherapy is ineffective; in that case, we can promptly substitute another, or if there is no alternative available, stop the treatment entirely. Thus situations in which an ineffective but toxic treatment is obstinately continued are either imaginary or the work of dangerous amateurs. The amateurs must be prevented from doing harm, but it is unfair to judge chemotherapy as a whole on the basis of their inept practice of it.

The loss of hair is another classic problem. In men, it is of only moderate importance, and besides—this is a fact that puzzles me but that all our patients have confirmed—the hair begins to grow back despite continuation of the treatment. In women, the loss of hair can be a very painful experience. It occurs in about 25 percent of cases, more often with certain cytostatics than with others. It is never permanent. Some of our patients wear wigs. They know that their hair will grow back. They also know that it would be dangerous to stop the treatment. But every year a few of our women patients slip through our fingers, in spite of our efforts to keep them, because they are beginning to lose their hair. It is true that for persons of a certain psychological makeup, such a change in self-image is unbearable. And often these are the very persons to whom it is impossible to reveal what is at stake in the battle being waged. We don't yet have a good means of overcoming the problem of hair loss. I shall merely point out to sympathetic souls that the permanent removal of a breast by extensive surgery is a mutilation that is at least equally traumatic. Why is it that the same persons who cheerfully prescribe or perform such surgery inveigh against chemotherapy, when chemotherapy is the very thing that promises to make it possible to perform smaller and smaller operations?

In recent years it has become fashionable to express concern about the quality of life. One has to have seen a cancer patient with disseminated lesions—a patient who is in constant pain despite analgesics that keep him only semiconscious—in order to realize how hypocritical it is to invoke the quality of life as an excuse for not treating. One has to have seen an effective chemotherapy, in which as soon as the treatment is started, the pain that would not yield to morphine diminishes or disappears for a period of a few weeks or even, as in many cases we have observed, for a period of years.

I therefore maintain that the pointless continuation of treatment— a practice rightly denounced by most members of the medical community—is not an inherent failing of palliative treatments for cancer. When it occurs, it is because the treatment was ill conceived or incorrectly applied or not indicated in the first place. Those who make such errors are solely responsible for them, and they don't reflect upon the collective effort of the professional chemotherapists.

By definition, in these situations of palliative treatment there comes a time when all hope of being effective disappears. At that point it would be absurd and cruel to continue a treatment that would add to the patient's suffering or even simply to his discomfort. Jean Bernard, Hamburger, Vic Dupont—outstanding physicians whose personal contributions in their respective fields have pushed back the frontiers of our effectiveness, that is, of our power to cure—have had excellent things to say on the subject of useless treatment and the doctor's responsibility when confronted with painful individual cases. Their wise, discriminating warnings have a very different ring from the statements of those who have never been personally involved—who have never allowed themselves to be personally involved—in these situations. And here, by the way, the first crack appears in our critics' façade of rationality and virtue.

I am perfectly willing to grant that gaining a few weeks in a situation of rapid spontaneous evolution isn't worth anything—unless the patient desires it. But now they are questioning the value of gaining months. May we ask how many months would have to be gained before they would deign to take an interest in a therapy? Eighteen? Twenty-four? Thirty-six? Would twelve months—even twelve months free from pain, at home, filled with hope—be too short a time for them? They condemn ineffective treatments, and rightly so, but the sleight of hand is to label ineffective any treatment that doesn't bring about permanent cure in 100 percent of cases. What about the kidney patients whose blood has to be purified artificially or who receive transplants, more and more of whom are being kept alive and active without any hope of ever being "cured," in the sense of being able to stop treatment? What would these patients have to say about the value of palliative treatments? What about the serious diabetics who depend on very burdensome treatments to keep them alive and active? What would they have to say on the subject?

Palliative treatments are considered valid for a whole series of diseases, but when it comes to cancer, it is all or nothing. Without asking the opinion of their patients, the extremists refuse to undertake any treatment unless it is sure to succeed; otherwise, morphine. They have a twofold argument: (a) *the treatments are dangerous* (which is meaningless unless one compares their dangers to those of the disease itself, and which in any event is based on now-outmoded practices); and (b) *the treatments are ineffective* (a judgment that can be made only if one has first defined the criteria of effectiveness for a wide variety of individual situations, which is not the case).

In the light of such an argument, to defend patients against these useless enterprises becomes an act of great and courageous humanism. And a doubt is left hovering about the reasons why certain doctors fight back: paranoia, vanity, careerism. For my part, I wonder about the reasons why certain doctors attack the efforts of the chemotherapists.

It's possible that everything is based on a misunderstanding. It is possible that they are willing to inform themselves, to read the regular issues of *Cancer, Cancer Treatment Reports, Cancer Research, Oncology, Medical and Pediatric Oncology,* the *Journal of Surgical Oncology, Cancer Treatment Reviews,* the *British Journal of Cancer,* the *International Journal of Cancer,* the *European Journal of Cancer,* the *Journal of the National Cancer Institute,* the *Bulletin du Cancer* (trust me, this is only a sampling). It's possible that when they come into contact with this avalanche of information, they will discover that they had a misconception about the situation. It's possible that they will then want to form a personal opinion, on the basis of this new information, and to find out whether it is true that they can improve their patients' chances without inflicting on them torments that they rightly dread.

But it's also possible that they will do nothing of the kind. It's possible—just a hypothesis—that they don't subscribe to the journals I have mentioned and that they will go on living on third-hand information that is ten years old. It's even possible that this refusal to inform themselves is not the result of laziness, but that it functions as an insurance against the risk of having to change their point of view. Why should all doctors be adults? By that I mean, among other things, persons who are able to give up ideas that are dear to them if reality demands it, without feeling thereby diminished. But we have not yet reached the heart of the matter. As I have said repeatedly throughout this book, cancer is a very special case. In our Western culture, this disease is unconsciously invested with a dimension of evil that sets it apart from all others. And there is absolutely no reason why doctors should be more likely than their patients to be able to communicate with their subconscious and become converts to rationality.

My thesis, in short, is that our "opponents" can't allow themselves to change their point of view, because they would have to settle certain difficult personal relations with death. Also, they would have to admit that the virtuous stand they have taken, their moral outrage, has served only to mask the existence of their own fear.

Psychiatrists tell us that a patient's illness reminds us of the possibility of our own illness, that the chance that the patient may die reminds us of our own mortality. Thus to take responsibility for the possible death of others is to be able to take responsibility for one's own. I believe this analysis is true. Many physicians have a horror of cancer because it is the unconscious image of their own death. And therefore, without realizing it, they have a horror of the patient who has cancer. They cut him off from the real world, they announce to the family that it's all over, that they must resign themselves to the inevitable, that no effort makes any sense. They will prescribe analgesics. But they won't commit themselves to a determined personal combat, because defeat would then be seen as their own defeat, the loss of the patient as their own loss, and that is something they can't bear. As I have said, relatives sometimes frankly confess to these terrors which physicians repress.

But this attitude doesn't apply to the first phase of treatment, the surgical phase, because surgery, which cuts and removes, is also, symbolically, a victorious act. That is why it would lose much of its value if one were to admit that a complementary treatment is necessary because there is a residual disease. And that is why many members of the medical community reject not only palliative treatments for tumors that have manifestly recurred but even potentially curative treatments for the postoperative disease that is still microscopic.

I would be unjust if I failed to mention that profound changes are taking place. Along with the "conservatives," young and old, who are frozen in an attitude of rejection, there are also numbers of physicians and surgeons, also of all ages, who even in the particular domain of cancer show themselves capable of abandoning their prejudices, overcoming their resistances, putting unhappy personal experiences in perspective and employing modern treatments. More and more patients are referred to us by physicians, surgeons, and radiologists who want to put the theses of the oncologists to an objective test, and who are prepared, if the test is positive, to reexamine their entire practice.

There are among them many practicing physicians who, as soldiers in the front lines, in contact with suffering, faced with families begging them to "do something," finally free themselves from the skepticism that was drilled into them. The urgent demands of their profession pierce the armor that was forged for them in medical school, and—I say it with no intent to flatter—it is to their honor that they are able to undo their training. There are also many professors, great consulting surgeons or physicians, who do the same, and it is even more to their credit, because they had been teaching the opposite. Their desire to serve the sick outweighs their prejudices. There are also men and women of such courage and integrity that their very existence should make us optimistic about the future of the species to which we belong.

This is not so surprising. More than any other profession, medicine, because of the immediacy of its sanctions, demands an open and objective mind and a readiness to make radical changes in one's point of view when the facts require it. One of the outstanding qualities of good doctors is precisely their ability to undertake this kind of intellectual operation, which is always difficult and always creates conflicts. That is why I'm not surprised to find that those whom I consider the best are willing, not to take our word for anything, we do not ask them to do that, but to put their opinions to the test. As for the others, I send the ball back into their court. It is up to them to explain themselves to their patients.

Let no one imagine that I am trying to drum up trade. At Lariboisière we receive five times as many patients as we should, given the means and space at our disposal. I should like nothing so much as to see more specialists being trained in cancer centers and university hospitals.

One more word, this time about nurses. Mine, who have agreed to share in our work, who grieve at our failures and rejoice in our successes, play a decisive role. They have managed to create a kindly and pleasant atmosphere in our chemotherapy unit that unquestionably helps to reassure the patients and their families and to de-dramatize and minimize side effects. But I know that they sometimes run into nurses from other units who, without having any first-hand experience, say to them, "What you are doing is a waste of time."

That is not all. The Welfare Administration is at last offering me a unit that is somewhat better adapted to our work, in another hospital. At present, it is used for general pulmonary diseases. Some nurses who have learned what it is to be used for in future have asked to be transferred to another ward. They too want to avoid having to face cancer patients. I don't blame them for it. They are reacting in the same way as most of our contemporaries.

At least I have the possibility of recruiting nurses who are motivated and therefore effective. My head nurse, whom I hope to be allowed to take with me, wonders whether some of our good results are not attributable to this motivation, to the general morale of our team. She may be right. While in theory our present procedures are capable of achieving a given level of success, it is clear that in practice much depends on the person who applies them. The doctor who "doesn't believe in it," and who uses the patient's fatigue as an excuse to stop a treatment after four months when it should last two years, will obviously have poorer results, which will in turn confirm his pessimism.

Part Five

✿✿✿

A GLANCE AT CLINICAL RESEARCH

I think I have shown that our present results are far better than they are generally thought to be, although unfortunately they are still restricted to a small number of patients. These results have been achieved in the course of a few years, by a few groups of doctors, who have had to brave abuse, silence, or ideological terrorism from the established teams in their respective countries. And they have been achieved despite the widespread belief that clinical research—research based on the observation of patients—is relatively unimportant at best and harmful at worst. A typical vicious circle, since to deprive clinical research of funds on the ground that it is worthless is to deny it the possibility of proving its worth. I want to open a debate within the debate by describing our problems, our tools, the methods we use. I have no intention of avoiding difficult questions, and I shall begin with the delicate problem of treatment trials.

14

❀❀❀

Treatment Trials

In discussing the therapeutic procedures available to us today and the various ways in which they are used, I have indicated that this or that treatment has been evaluated and credited with a given result. I have also shown where my own preferences lie, on the basis of the studies that have already been carried out, and which new studies I would like to see given priority. But—and this point is crucial—I'm not trying to convince anyone of the superior logic of my view or the view of the groups with which I work. On the contrary, we have had quite enough of logic, of deductive, Cartesian medicine, of brilliant intuitions and "impressions" based on a practice that rules out all criticism. The only thing that counts is real progress, the objective proof that procedure B is 10 percent more effective than procedure A and should be substituted for it (if, and only if, what is gained in quantity is not lost in quality). Or that, contrary to favorable "impressions," it is 10 percent less effective and should be abandoned.

Most people have no idea what a fantastic risk of error they are running when, in all good faith, they allow themselves to form an impression. (I have forbidden my students to say, "I have the impression that he is better," or "I have the impression that this treatment is more active.") It is perfectly true that when penicillin was made available to clinicians, they found out immediately, after treating only a handful of cases, that the drug cured the most serious septicemias and contagious diseases, which otherwise proved fatal within a few days. But it was much harder to establish that this same penicillin was active against syphilis, a chronic disease, and that streptomycin could change the formerly inevitable course of tubercular meningitis. With regard to cancers, what we are trying to establish today is not yet, unfortunately, that a given drug cures 100 percent of cases in two weeks, but that administered over a period of two years, the drug improves by 80, 60, or even 20 percent the rate of five-year survival in a given situation. And that the improvement occurs under conditions that the statisticians consider "significant"—that is, such that there is less than a 5 percent risk of attributing to the treatment a difference that is in reality the result of chance.

It is impossible to establish the reality of these differences on the basis of one's impressions. An impression derived from twenty consecutive patients can prove radically false if the study is continued on two hundred patients. It could be the result of chance, or of the fact that those twenty patients had very special characteristics that made them particularly responsive to the treatment, while others don't benefit from it. But once Dr. X has formed a favorable impression, every patient he treats thereafter will be given—in all good faith—an ineffective treatment, which will simultaneously deprive him of other treatments that are really active. And if Dr. X has any gift for public relations and intellectual terrorism, not only his patients but countless others as well will take the wrong road—still in all good faith.

At this point, the only thing we can do is conduct rigorous therapeutic trials designed in such a way that we can reach objective truth—with less than 5 percent risk of error. It is therefore better to discuss frankly the problems posed by such trials and the methods that cancer specialists have developed to try to solve them. I shall explain those methods in detail. But before I begin, let me say that any help or suggestions, as opposed to negative criticism, will be welcome. If the public considers that the problem of drug trials and treatment trials is too serious to be left to the physicians, let the public intervene. Let joint groups be formed to discuss the ways in which they should be conducted, and even to draw up rules. But I must insist that it is one thing to improve the techniques of trials, and another to reject trials entirely. If the patients of 1978 don't want to be the subjects of trials, they must resign themselves to being treated as they would have been in 1968. That may not be important in a case of eczema, but to a patient with a cancer, it may mean the difference between life and death. No doubt that is why the methodology of therapeutic trials was first developed by doctors working with cancer.

Let us salute in passing the host of oncologists who work on animal models. I shall not go into detail about these trials, which are very complex and highly codified. But the reader should know that in the various laboratories of the U.S. National Cancer Institute, 50,000 different compounds are tested every year, which represents an incalculable service to the entire human species. And as soon as a product from another country is announced as being potentially active, the NCI uses its extensive laboratory facilities to test that product again and send the results to the author, without deriving the least financial benefit or scientific credit from this work. A system of animal tumor models makes it possible to identify more than 80 percent of products that have a chance of being active in human beings. The others are tested separately. As soon as any agent is identified as being potentially effective—even if no one has the least idea of the way it works—it is subjected to toxicity trials in large animals and to pharmacological studies. The maximum dose tolerated by animals is determined, and the relation between that dose and the effective dose; a great variety of tumors are tested, and the final step is to manufacture by small-scale methods a sufficient quantity of the pure product. At this point, the experimenters turn to the clinicians.

When a drug has never been used on human beings before, the clinicians begin with phase I trials: however fascinating the experimental results may have been, the doctors to whom the drug is entrusted will handle it like an explosive. Indeed, they can't be certain of either its effectiveness or its toxicity, because the notable differences between species make it impossible to extrapolate from experimental observations. All they know is that there is a chance that the product will be effective and a strong possibility that its toxicity won't be prohibitive. This last point is the first to be checked. How and on whom? The present rules laid down by the National Cancer Institute—so far as I know, no one has yet laid down any such rules in France, but some are being studied—provide that the initial dose of the product will be one-third, by kilo of body weight or by square meter of body surface, of the maximum dose tolerated by the animal having the lowest tolerance. Thereafter, the dose is systematically and carefully escalated, according to the method devised by Leonardo Fibonacci and modified by my friend Oleg Selawry of Miami. Thus, little by little, the physicians arrive at an estimate of the maximum dose that can be given without severe or lasting side effects, and also an estimate of the time that should elapse between two successive doses.

But who are the subjects of these trials? They are patients with tumors that are not only advanced but also resistant to all available treatments, the various procedures having been tried unsuccessfully either on the patient in question or on similar cases. Furthermore, in the United States, where these trials take place, the law requires that the patient sign a statement of "informed consent." One may wonder just how "informed" such consent can really be, but it means that the physician is not at any rate playing hide-and-seek with his patient. I shall go into this thorny problem at length later. The results of the phase I trials, which are entrusted to a few hand-picked teams, are published, along with all the conclusions regarding precautions to be taken in using the drug and any observations as to its effectiveness. But it's generally understood that effectiveness may have been underestimated, because the product was tried on patients in an advanced stage of the disease, and that in such cases a halt in growth of the tumor is equivalent to a regression in a smaller tumor or one that isn't evolving so rapidly.

Next come the phase II trials. The drug is supplied to more teams for a first real evaluation of its effectiveness, both at the maximum dose tolerated by human beings and also at lesser doses (administered, for example, at shorter intervals). The goal is to explore as wide a range of tumors as possible, so as to discover which cases might benefit most from the treatment in the future. The phase II trials usually require the cooperation of a large number of teams. Naturally, these trials are also carried out on patients who can't be successfully treated in any other way and who, in the United States, give their informed consent. Here again, the normal obligation to propose the new treatment only to patients at a very advanced stage is likely to cause the effectiveness of the procedure to be underestimated. But at least the dose used is the maximum, and it is applied to as great a variety of cases as possible.

One might think that different teams using the same criteria of response—those described in the chapter on chemotherapy—would arrive at comparable results. Yet on reading the specialized literature and the tables constantly distributed by the NCI, one is struck by the fact that the number of responses can range from 10 to 80 percent. How are we to explain such a discrepancy? It is caused in part by the varying degrees of enthusiasm of the different investigators—that is, by the element of subjectivity, which the most rigorous methods of clinical evaluation can't entirely eliminate. It is also caused by the great differences between one group of patients and another. This is a key point. Very large numbers are required in order to obtain reasonable certainties. If three lung cancers are included in a phase II trial, two of which respond to the treatment, it by no means follows that the product tested is effective in two-thirds of cases. It may be that in a series of twenty, these two cases will be the only ones to respond.

Generally, the NCI's Division of Cancer Treatment, whose director is Vincent DeVita, Jr., compiles an average of the results reported by the different groups, tumor by tumor, and considers an agent to have been evaluated when it has been used on at least a hundred comparable cases. When the average number of responses is less than 15 percent, the drug is considered ineffective for the site studied. That often happens, and it means that not all the agents the laboratory people place at our disposal are used to treat human beings. This policy is perhaps too conservative. Some products prove to be highly toxic. Many are wholly ineffective, or only marginally effective. Nevertheless, there are occasional surprises. A product that has been declared ineffective, when reevaluated later by other groups with different modalities of administration (for example, distribution of the dose over a perfusion of twenty-four hours or over five consecutive days), sometimes proves capable of producing regressions.

All is now ready for the final stage of the study, the phase III trials. These are conducted on patients with disseminated but "new" (previously untreated) tumors, selected among the categories that showed the greatest sensitivity in the phase II trials. At this stage it is possible to evaluate the drug with relative precision, and under the best conditions for effectiveness. But the investigators responsible for these trials are obsessed by the risk that they will conclude *mistakenly* that the drug is effective and thereby set therapeutic efforts on the wrong track for years to come. Twenty percent of partial regressions in an isolated series doesn't mean much. It could, as I said, be the result of chance or of a particularly favorable distribution of the cases in the series. That is why it has been agreed to compare the treatment under study to the best treatment already available, and a series of procedures have been established for this purpose.

"Randomization"—the drawing of patients by lot, according to very strict rules—is necessary to ensure the comparability of the groups receiving treatment A and treatment B. As recently as fifteen years ago, the drug to be tested was generally compared to an inactive product, a placebo, because the agents then available had such a low level of effectiveness: the investigators had to make sure that the results they observed couldn't have been due to an accident of the tumor's spontaneous evolution. That's no longer the case today. A phase III trial includes a control group, which the international chemotherapy associations periodically attempt to standardize, and which consists of a group of patients who receive the proven therapeutic agent that is considered most active.

Whenever it is possible to do so, the patients are first divided into subgroups according to prognosis. This is a way of ensuring, without resorting to enormous numbers of cases, that when the two groups to be compared are chosen at random, members of the various subgroups will be equally distributed between them. It may be that the treatment is active only in one subgroup, a fact that it would be essential not to miss.

"Crossing over," a special design often used for a phase III trial, provides that in case one of the two treatments fails, either initially or because there is a later relapse, the other will be substituted for it. In this way, the doctors hope to learn whether or not the two treatments have a cross resistance, a piece of information that is crucial for the elaboration of combinations.

It is generally provided that only a fixed number of patients will be drawn by lot for a given series of phase III trials. This number is calculated by the biostatisticians of the NCI and the cooperative groups, or by those at the headquarters of the EORTC (European Organization for Research on the Treatment of Cancer) in Brussels and on the team of Professors Schwartz and Flamant in Villejuif. It is done in such a way as to minimize the possibility that a difference between the two groups studied will go unnoticed if it is only moderate. Slowly the results are compiled. The observations on all cases are checked—my associates and I spend hours at this every week—and finally the statisticians calculate the probability that the difference recorded is attributable to chance.

If the probability is less than 5 percent, and by virtue of a solid agreement among biostatisticians the world over, *only* if that is the case, the difference is considered attributable to the effectiveness of the product. We can then see if treatment B is superior to treatment A, if its mechanism of action is different in principle and if its toxicity is acceptable. Obviously a treatment that is inferior to the one used as a control but that has low toxicity and a different mechanism of action won't be rejected. In principle, a reliable phase III study will determine its place in the arsenal for the cancer community as a whole.

Needless to say, the reason why all these studies are necessary is that the differences are slight—that is, each agent is still only relatively effective. Let me repeat: the day we run across a "penicillin" for cancer that makes 98 percent of tumors disappear in a week, we will not need all this apparatus to recognize its effectiveness. At the moment, we aren't in that position. The percentages of effectiveness are rising slowly but surely, and it is the studies described here that have enabled us, from year to year, to select the best treatments.

The evaluation of combinations of drugs has given rise to a curious phenomenon in the last few years. Effective cytostatic agents have been "coming out" so fast that it hasn't been possible to try their various combinations in a rational way. Today there are more than forty effective cytostatics. To test all their possible combinations, two by two, three by three, and so on, would require a fabulous number of trials, and we would have to give up testing the new drugs that came out in the meantime. But the chemotherapists, and the statisticians who advise them, are only beginning to recognize this fact. For years, most of them have refused—quite unreasonably, in my opinion—to take any interest in combinations of three drugs so long as all the combinations of two have not been tested. In 1965, when I published my first studies of an empirical but effective combination of five cytostatic agents, no one was prepared to grant that it was a good way to proceed. Li's work with three drugs in 1960 had not been taken seriously, nor had Greenspan's in 1962. Today it is acceptable for clinicians to study combinations before all the intermediary stages have been completed. In principle, their methods are less empirical than they used to be, but in working out new combinations they are often guided by simple reasoning rather than by the subtle and problematical concepts of experimental chemotherapy.

Certain phase III trials are comparing the results of a combination of three or four drugs to those of a single agent. And on the day, already in the distant past, when Vincent DeVita and Paul Carbone perfected the combination of four drugs known as M.O.P.P. for Hodgkin's disease—a condition I haven't spoken of because it lies within the competence of the hematologists—the results were so much better than anything that had been seen before that the purists had to give in and agree that from then on M.O.P.P. would be the standard to which all new treatments for Hodgkin's disease would be compared. Jean Bernard's team took M.O.P.P. as a point of departure for their important work in this field.

The evaluation of combined approaches is an absolute nightmare for the statisticians because it involves a series of parameters and concepts that they have not yet really worked out and that they are reluctant to deal with. For example, the response will not be obtained in all cases at the same stage of treatment. Step 2 won't start at the same time in all patients, because that will depend on the response to step 1. And so on. In such a situation there are two possible reactions: the reaction of the bureaucrat, who forbids such trials or refuses to consider them (and from this point of view there are as many bureaucrats in the American cooperative groups as elsewhere); and the reaction of the uninhibited biostatistician, who will find the statistical apparatus he needs in order to analyze the results of such a study. The patients' interest is the prime consideration, but that simple fact is not always obvious to everyone.

•　　•　　•

Clearly, the very existence of trials raises grave problems that are not merely technical but ethical in nature, problems that haven't always been solved and that I have no wish to evade. I want to examine them from the only point of view that really matters: at a time when available treatments are not considered satisfactory, and when new treatments and new concepts are constantly emerging, how can we protect the true interests of the patients?

Is it possible *not* to conduct trials? I confess that I don't see how. If I have a treatment for advanced lung cancers that gives a rate of response of 30 percent, and if I hope that by combining it with, or preceding it by, a new procedure, I can increase the chances of response, how can I not try? Future results will be, like present results, the fruit of an uninterrupted series of trials. Without going into all the technical reasons, I repeat that animal experiments, which are always necessary, can be only partially extrapolated to human beings. But I also want to emphasize that not everything is permissible. Charlatans conduct trials absolutely at random—and no one criticizes them for it.

We doctors who do clinical research, taking the best advantage we can of the fragmentary facts that we establish or that others establish for us while we wait for the princes of basic research to find a cure for our patients, would fail in our duty if we did not conduct trials. The application of M.O.P.P., which transformed the prognosis for Hodgkin's disease, was a trial. So were the successful reinduction treatments for acute leukemia, proposed by Jean Bernard, and the immunotherapy of acute leukemia during periods of remission, proposed by Mathé.

Members of the public sometimes say that patients in hospitals are used as guinea pigs. That is clearly unfair, because the goal of the doctors who treat them is to use the trials to improve the individual fate of the patients who place themselves in their hands. But in any event, the fundamental concept of therapeutic trials can't be rejected unless we are willing to call a halt to all medical progress. And naturally it is in hospitals, and not in private consulting rooms, that such studies can be carried out: different specialists must pool their skills; nurses and secretaries must contribute long hours of work; laboratory equipment must be available, as well as extensive records and statistics. Fortunately, with the financial assistance of the administration and of Social Security, this work continues to be carried out in our hospitals, and that is one reason why there are many medical specialties in which French contributions are internationally recognized.

The drawing of patients by lot raises a very delicate question that can generally be counted on to divide any medical assembly into two fiercely opposed camps. One evening in the United States, at the annual dinner of one of the cooperative groups, I was vehemently taken to task by an eminent biostatistician who had an important position with the NCI, because I had published a chemotherapy study that did not include a "randomized" control group. His argument ran as follows: "In carrying out and publishing a study that you think is positive and that was not controlled according to the internationally accepted rules, you have been guilty of a real crime against the community of future patients. For one thing, you've been willing to form an opinion based on impressions, memories, unreliable comparisons. And now that you are convinced, you would think it unethical to turn back and treat your patients as you did before. Therefore, you are condemning the patients who are entrusted to you in the future to undergo a treatment that has no guarantee and that may be inferior to the preceding one. But the worst of it is that if you are right, and other chemotherapists do not follow you—because we have trained them well—then you are depriving all their patients of an advance. And all because you didn't take the trouble to convince others according to the scientific norms, by means of a randomization between the patients who received your treatment and those in your control series."

But many a time, when I have tried to persuade my compatriots of this sort of viewpoint, they have criticized me just as bluntly. "How could you," they say, "a physician in whom a given patient has placed his confidence, who is supposed to advise him conscientiously, according to the best of your experience—how could you have the audacity to decide what treatment to recommend to him by drawing lots? It would be a betrayal of trust. I pity the American patients!" I think that pretty well sums up the debate. On one side are the rigid scientists who consider that the clinician's "impressions" have already done enough harm, and that in the interest of the patients it is time to rely on the strict evidence of facts and figures. On the other side are the physicians who were trained in humanism before they were trained in the discipline of research and statistics. They take the chance of making a mistake, but they want to play their role of private counselor to the end. Is it possible to combine the advantages of both attitudes and eliminate the disadvantages?

Some concrete examples will help to clarify the debate. In Europe, the EORTC is currently conducting a trial on lung cancer in which the control group is given no treatment whatever after the operation. In other words, the control group is following the advice given the vast majority of patients by surgeons who reject trials. The purpose of this is to try to answer the following questions:

Is something added by radiotherapy? No one knows for certain. Some think radiation is beneficial, others that it is bad because of its effect on immunity.

Is something added by chemotherapy, both for patients who have had radiation and for those who haven't? Almost all surgeons consider it harmful. Some consider it necessary. As I have said, a Japanese team has just published surprising results, but without a control series, and in contradiction to other studies.

Is something added by immunotherapy, both for patients who have had radiation and for those who haven't? Is it possible, for example, that immunotherapy cancels out the potentially harmful effects of radiation, thereby making the beneficial effects appear more plainly? No one has yet given a clear answer to this question.

Lastly, is something added by a combination of chemotherapy and immunotherapy, both after radiation and in the absence of radiation?

The truth is that the answers to these questions aren't known. That being the case, the conservatives choose abstention, on the ground that postoperative treatments may be harmful. The enthusiasts choose treatment, on the ground that for the past twenty years there has been no progress in the statistics on surgery. Each faction publishes its results, but no one is convinced. If the enthusiasts report an improvement of 25 percent, the conservatives reply that it is an accidental series, probably "skewed" by unconscious selection, and that they themselves could report comparable results recently achieved on short series by surgery alone. Here their own argument turns against them. For if they don't consider the reported improvement convincing, it is because it lacks what might have made it convincing: a control series rendered completely comparable to the test series by strict randomization. But the moment they refuse this randomization, they condemn their patients to undergo the "old" treatment for a long time, until the difference announced is not 25 percent but 100 percent. There are situations in which it is really impossible to tell in advance whether or not an added treatment will be beneficial. Often its effect won't be spectacular, and the only way to determine that it is useful is to make a strict comparison according to the rules of statistics. In these situations, those who refuse to include their patients in a therapeutic trial involving randomization may have to take the responsibility for causing our knowledge, and hence our power, to stagnate for a long time. They prefer to display before their patients an assurance that in reality they don't—or shouldn't—feel. Thus they preserve an image of themselves that gives them a clear conscience, to which they may not be entitled.

On the other hand, it is possible to resist the tyranny of the biostatisticians, not in such a way as to refuse progress, but so as to make progress under conditions that are less rigid and, I think, more equitable. Because these gentlemen are indeed tyrannical. When one says to them, "Here are my results with lung cancers in 1975 as compared to my results in 1972; the probability that the difference between them is due to chance is insignificant," they reply, "You have no right to calculate that probability. The two series to which you refer weren't made comparable by randomization. Furthermore, you have no guarantee that lung cancer in 1975 is the same disease as lung cancer in 1972. Consequently, you have no right to compare treatment B of 1975 with treatment A of 1972. You have to start over again every year with a randomization between A and B, or A and C, or B and C."

For a long time this sort of argument triumphed and all protest was silenced. But at last open rebellion has been declared, thanks to the courage of Freireich and Gehan, an American team at M. D. Anderson Institute in Houston. These investigators base their comparisons on "historical controls"—that is, old cases matched to the new ones by as many characteristics as possible. They refuse to randomize—that is, to assign some of their patients to the control treatment when they think they have something better to offer. The whole cancer community is closely following this battle, in which the two champions of the new cause have already suffered some blows. Clearly, it is hard to come to a conclusion, and deciding absolutely in favor of one attitude or the other won't help to advance matters. I admit—and I am going against the statistics "craze" in France and elsewhere—that I think the position of Freireich and Gehan is the best (or the least bad) at the present time. What I can't abide is taking the absence of scientific rigor as an excuse to do nothing, to favor the status quo, when progress could be made. But that is precisely what both parties are doing in this case. The French surgeons, like certain biostatisticians of the NCI, prefer to stick to treatments of the past that may be outmoded. Some of them feel this way because they haven't been deeply, personally convinced; others because they would rather commit hara-kiri than be deeply, personally convinced when the rules of the statistical game haven't been followed. One solution might be to use "historical controls" that would be very carefully chosen, and perhaps chosen by persons other than the investigators. That might be a way of breaking out of the present paralysis, while still respecting both the rights of every patient and the demands of the science that serves him—and without which any help he receives is only a deception.

One reason why there is so much controversy over clinical trials is that our knowledge and techniques are still inadequate. The situation will soon be clarified as we make progress, especially with regard to the rapid evaluation of treatments.

I can already cite one example of such progress from my own work on measurable lung tumors. We have been able to establish that when the rate of growth of a tumor is known, we have only to find out its response to two consecutive chemotherapy injections to be able to predict what will happen. By feeding a simple mathematical model into a desk-top computer, we are able to tell after one month of a treatment whether or not it will be useful to prolong it. Thus in cases of measurable tumors, we can evaluate treatments very quickly, gaining considerable time for the patient. If he is not one of those who will benefit from the treatment tried, we discover it almost immediately and move on to a different treatment.

I am trying to persuade the Eastern Cooperative Oncology Group to treat these categories of patients separately, so as to accelerate our evaluation procedures. I must say that so far I've tried in vain. Innovations are considered suspect on both sides of the Atlantic. The reason

I'm pressing the Americans is that they have the structures for coopera-tion that we lack. The day they agree, a hundred centers will test our proposal. Here in France, we don't yet have anything similar, and only individual studies are likely to see the light.

Another way of making evaluation procedures more flexible might be to agree that in a randomized trial the statisticians wouldn't deter-mine in advance the number of patients necessary for the correct interpretation of results. Instead, they would constantly compare the profiles of the test series and the control series and announce any divergence as soon as it appeared. It seems there are mathematical arguments against such a procedure, and they have been published. I didn't understand them, which takes nothing away from their validity. But I believe it is time for the biostatisticians to admit that they owe us more sophisticated tools and more flexible procedures. Fifteen years ago the problem was to find out if a given treatment was worth some-thing rather than nothing. Usually it was worth nothing. It was neces-sary to lay down rigid rules in order to guard against premature enthusi-asm, especially on the part of those incorrigible Europeans. Today the problem is to find out if we have made a genuine gain of 5 percent, and to find it out as soon as possible, so that as soon as possible, all patients can have the benefit of the improvement.

While respecting the prime concern of objectivity, we must lighten our machinery of evaluation. Some physicist friends of mine who are working in the field of high energy use ultra-sophisticated methods for calculating the probabilities of rare events. Would it not be possible to extrapolate those techniques to our situation? Perhaps they would en-able us to evaluate on the basis of a small number of cases, but still scientifically, the probability that a given treatment X is superior to treatment Y.

But how do we know that in the midst of all these technical debates, doctors won't lose sight of the interests of the individual patient—the patient who is suddenly thrust into the center of the scientific enter-prise by personal tragedy? This is a very serious problem. I have con-demned a reactionary attitude toward treatment, but I freely admit that overenthusiasm can be equally dangerous. Today it is no longer possible to leave the design of certain trials solely to the initiative of a given team: there are too many risks involved. One is that the patient

may be made to incur real dangers for the sake of a benefit that is likely
to be small, if not illusory. Another risk, and a terrible one, is that some
physicians, allowing their scientific curiosity to get the better of their
desire to be of service here and now, may try to discover only facts of
a fundamental nature without any immediate application to therapy.
That is really what patients are referring to when they protest against
the idea of being used as guinea pigs. I think I can state that this risk
is infinitesimal, at least in the area that I'm concerned with. But
infinitesimal is still too great. It must be reduced to zero.

A number of solutions to this problem have been devised in the
United States. All treatment protocols must be approved by the National Cancer Institute; in each hospital they must be approved by an
ethics committee having authority over all departments; finally, each
patient must sign a declaration of "informed consent" to participate
in the trial. There are almost no comparable structures in France.

This brings us to the final problem, that of "informed consent."
Every time I take part in cooperative studies within the ECOG, I am
asked for the written consent of my patients. Every time I explain that
because of cultural differences, I don't feel I have the right to ask for
such consent, as this would presuppose that whatever the circumstances, the raw truth should be revealed to the patient. But I admit
that I'm beginning to be contaminated by this requirement. I'm well
aware that consent of this sort can never really be informed. For one
thing, the patient is necessarily subjective: he can't possibly make a
decision as if the problem didn't concern him. For another, it is impossible for us to evaluate the results of a given method precisely in
advance and to answer the patient's questions on the level that matters
to him. But I'm also gradually coming to realize that our working rules
should be modified and that we should rely on other authorities besides
our own sense of responsibility. It is not good for a doctor to be a judge
—or sole judge, at any rate—in his own case. I look forward to the day
when we can appear before an ethics committee, so as to have a better
chance of making a wise decision on the design of a new study, and
also to the day when we can communicate with our patients on a deeper
level and with a greater degree of truth. I have often been present, in
various American hospitals, at the conversation that leads to the patient's signing of his "informed consent." What the patient usually says

is, "Do whatever you think is best, Doctor. I trust you." Often he signs
without having inquired into the real problems raised by the trial in
which the doctor is going to have him participate. He knows instinc-
tively that the fundamental concern of those who worked out the
structure of the trial was to protect his interests, so far as possible given
present knowledge. Even if the patient's acquiescence may seem superficial, I think it makes the relationship between him and his doctor
infinitely more honest and straightforward, and also more humane.

15

❀❀❀

Clinical Research

I know that many readers of this book will accuse me of being overoptimistic about the results that can be expected in the near future from clinical research. First, because cancer, like syphilis thirty years ago, can not be cured. Second, because the tendencies toward improvement of results are recent, and they are not evident to outside observers. A few years ago, much publicity was given in France to an article by an American journalist, Greenberg. After analyzing current American statistics, Greenberg wrote that from 1950 to 1969 the number of patients who survived for five years had increased by only 5 percent on the average. He even gave examples of cancers for which the survival rates were lower in 1969 than they were in 1950. Throughout this book I have tried to show that, despite the absence of support, applied research has made important progress. Thus there appears to be an irreconcilable contradition between my thesis and Greenberg's. But I think this contradiction can be explained.

Greenberg based his analysis entirely on the results of the treatments of 1969, available five years later in 1974, and he based it on the total results of the United States as a whole, including those obtained by the most traditional practices of the time.

For example, he says that from 1959 to 1969 the rate of survival of patients with breast cancers advanced by only 4 percent, in spite of the much-talked-about development of treatments combining surgery, radiation, and drugs. There is a major error here. Combined treatments may have been much talked about, but no breast-cancer patient treated in 1969 received drugs in the postoperative period. The five-year results of Fisher and Carbone's trials won't be available until 1979, and even then they will be drowned in the mass of results of conventional treatments prescribed throughout the United States as a whole. Yet after nearly three years their results already reveal a very important advance. These results are decisive, not only for breast cancers but for the very concept of postoperative adjuvant chemotherapy as a prophylaxis against metastases. They have stimulated various sectors, and other teams throughout the world have set to work following their lead.

Greenberg won't perceive the results until 1980, but there are many of us who can already declare, on the basis of results we have obtained at two years or even one year, that the progress is certain. Furthermore, as I have explained at length, the combined approaches are useful in inoperable cases as well. And lastly, it must be remembered that several active chemotherapeutic agents that are now used to combat solid tumors didn't exist in 1969, nor did certain effective procedures for stimulating immunity.

I shall not speak about fundamental research, because I am not competent to do so, but it has obviously taken giant steps. As for clinical research, it has been developing very rapidly, if I may judge from my own experience in one of the five great American cooperative groups sponsored and funded by the National Cancer Institute.

In 1970, at the Cancer Congress in Houston, I met two American colleagues who had each done me the honor of coming to see me in Paris. Their interest had been aroused by some articles I had published —which, by the way, it was much to their credit to have found and deciphered in French medical journals. These men told me that they were both members of the Eastern Cooperative Oncology Group, which in principle brings together all the great departments of general or specialized oncology on the East Coast, from Boston to Miami. I asked them if it would be possible for me to join them, because I was impatiently seeking structures for cooperative research that are still cruelly lacking in France. I was told that they would present my candidacy, but that there might be a problem about admitting a foreigner.

Goldin, with whom I was in correspondence, supported my candidacy with the new chairman of the group, Paul Carbone, and I was invited to participate in its work for a one-year probationary period. During that time I would be expected to take part in working out treatment protocols and in studying the effects of those (and only those) to which I had agreed. Also, I would have to attend the three annual meetings of the group, each of which lasts two and a half days. On the recommendation of the then Minister of Foreign Affairs, Maurice Schumann, the Ministry's Office of Scientific Affairs agreed to provide the necessary airplane tickets and since then has given me consistent support for which I am most grateful. Without it, these working relations couldn't have been established.

I did my best to perfect my English so that I would be able to follow rapid discussions and to defend a point of view against persons who would not hesitate to contradict me. And gradually I discovered how the group functions. For almost every type of cancer there is a different committee, presided over by a chairman who changes every two years. For every clinical situation within each type, there is a different treatment protocol, proposed by one of the members of the group and adopted, after having been shuttled back and forth, sometimes for a long time, between the author, the NCI, the chairman, and all the members of the group. Once it is adopted, several copies of the protocol, a detailed document of some fifteen pages, are sent to each member. Each member is requested, without obligation, to treat appropriate patients according to the modalities thus laid down. The patients are given weekly examinations, and very thorough monthly examinations, and reports are made on special forms and sent regularly to the secretariat of the group.

My student and friend Alain Depierre, assistant professor at Lariboisière, spends dozens of hours of overtime every month on this record-keeping, without which our results would remain unusable. The statistical center at Buffalo, which has a knowledgeable and well-equipped staff, examines the data sheets, asks for additional information, and picks up errors or omissions. At each meeting of the group there is a progress report on each protocol, followed by discussion. As soon as a conclusion has been reached, the protocol is withdrawn and replaced by another, which builds on the results of the first. The group brings together more than forty departments of medical oncology, and their cooperative effort is so powerful that they can find in twelve to eighteen months answers that a single investigator working alone would need a lifetime to obtain. Furthermore, when protocols call for the use of drugs that have been developed by the NCI but are not yet available commercially, those drugs are sent free to participating institutions, including Lariboisière.

The advantages of this type of organization are obvious, and I shall not belabor them. Of course, there are disadvantages as well. One is that it generally takes the agreement of the majority of the group to put a protocol into operation, and, naturally, it is easier to obtain such agreement on concepts that are the least aggressive and most acceptable at the time they are proposed. That is why many of the great revolutions in treatment are carried out by small teams conducting pilot studies rather than by the cooperative groups, which are more interested in "holding the ground." Another disadvantage lies in the fact that, because of their composition, these groups are more inclined to study a single modality of treatment—chemotherapy—than combined approaches. In order to explore the latter, they would first have to organize meetings of surgeons and radiologists and convince them of the need for collaboration. But the NCI's Division of Cancer Treatment, under the leadership of DeVita and Muggia, is making a great effort to get the cooperative groups to give priority to studies of combined strategies, and especially of postoperative immunochemotherapies.

One of the basic functions of the cooperative groups is to confirm the pilot studies of their members or of other teams. As I said in the chapter on trials, one good result out of a series of twenty cases is of only limited significance. Neither cancer specialists nor their patients are interested in an investigator's being able to plume himself on extraordinary results (which are usually overestimated). What they *are* interested in is being able to determine the real extent of those results, to find out whether they can be reproduced, and to measure exactly their possible cost in toxicity. The NCI will not endorse a study unless it can be checked by one of the cooperative groups or "task forces" sponsored by the Institute. And for this purpose it supplies the neces-

sary funds, allocated by the state and the Congress. If results that have
been published abroad seem promising, it will undertake to have them
checked as well. It goes to great lengths to verify reported progress. In
1969, when Cooper published his results on disseminated breast cancers (more than 85 percent of "responses" to a combination of four
drugs), the NCI dispatched a three-member commission to investigate.
The commission asked to see all the data and all the patients and then
publicly disputed Cooper's results, saying they were much too optimistic. (They were indeed, but less so than the commission thought. A
controversy began that was to last three or four years before there was
agreement on the real rate of response: around 65 percent, which is
already excellent and has since been exceeded.)

Thus, research on treatment is—and should be—carried out primarily in the form of cooperative studies, within groups specifically designed for the purpose. But clearly, research on treatment is not everything. Several times I have mentioned in passing other subjects that can
be studied only by clinicians. Animal diseases are very different from
clinical situations. The immunologic conditions governing the rejection of a cancer can't possibly be the same in a human being with a
spontaneous tumor as in a specially bred mouse with a tumor that has
been transplanted for generations. The time that elapses between onset
of the disease and treatment is entirely different in human beings and
in laboratory animals. So are the risks incurred in treatment. (For
instance, the doses of immunostimulant we usually apply to human
beings are a hundred times lower than those we use with experimental
animals.)

In short, the two situations are never the same but only analogous.
Therefore, while we can still expect enormous progress to come out of
experimental studies, we will really learn to cure human cancers only
by studying and treating them where they appear. For example, with
the help of Dr. Peltier, research director at INSERM, who has kindly
agreed to examine blood samples from my patients, I am collecting data
on changes in the blood complement system, changes that vary from
case to case and must be corrected individually. Such data cannot be
extrapolated from studies of animals.

This is only one example out of a thousand showing that the clinical
investigator is an essential link in the chain that will lead to success.

By forcing him to analyze the obstacles he meets, his profession leads him to ask questions that would never occur to an experimental oncologist, much less to a molecular biologist. Usually he does not have the necessary expertise to answer these questions himself, and therein lies another problem: he must find an interlocutor, and that is not easy, for every experimenter has his own program, his own priorities, his own ideas.

It is here that the flexibility and mobility of the Americans are probably most important. In the United States, a clinician's career is not necessarily fixed. If he has a plan for a coherent research program, he submits it to the National Cancer Institute. He receives in the form of grants the money needed to carry it out and hires the necessary medical and laboratory personnel for the agreed-upon period. If the program calls for heavy equipment that he lacks, he may use the grant to purchase it or even to have appropriate accommodations built to house it.

The problem now, in my opinion, is that working alone, the United States will not be able to resolve the last difficulties in a short time. As I have often said to my colleagues of the NCI, putting men on the moon was a feat within the capability of NASA, but moving from 40 percent success in the treatment of cancer to 80 percent in the next decade demands cooperation, coordination, and a distribution of tasks on not a national level but an international one. For the last two years I've been working, along with others, to institutionalize cooperation between France and the United States in clinical research related to concrete objectives, not to fundamental principles. Apparently that is much more difficult than I would have thought, and the difficulties have for a long time been all on the French side. But at last it is being done. Otherwise, France would be absent from the movement which leading developed nations are already joining in, a movement of true international cooperation and not of sterile competition.

Conclusion

In a world ruled by logic and reason, cancer would occupy the same place in the collective consciousness as the other potentially fatal diseases. The "basic" sciences would study its causes, its mechanisms, and the sovereign means of curing it, and doctors would use the knowledge gained to draw up plans of treatment. Controversies would never become emotional. Facts would be accepted by everyone, and wouldn't be interpreted in contradictory ways.

Clearly, we are not living in a logical, rational world. A debate often involves something much more than—and sometimes very different from—the search for truth. The history of medicine is particularly rich in examples of stormy controversy, and discussions of medical matters today reflect the general increase in aggressiveness, irrationality, and obscurantism. So I am well aware that the theses of this book will meet with determined and indignant adversaries. That doesn't concern me greatly. The important thing is that these theses should be known and debated by the interested parties, and that an examination of the facts should lead to changes in old practices.

I have tried to show in this book that real knowledge acquired in recent years, operational knowledge about the treatment of cancer, is denied, and that most patients are treated as if it hadn't been acquired.

One reason for this is that the knowledge was acquired in an "impure," empirical, disorderly fashion, while the fundamental cause of cancer is still not understood. Personally, I must say that that doesn't disturb me. The term "basic" has always seemed to me to be inappropriate to describe sciences that do not lie at the base of the edifice but rather crown its summit. No one takes exception to the fact that the experimental physicists have recently discovered scores of particles, while the theoreticians still can't say what matter is made of. And long before that, they exploded their bomb.

When it comes to treating disease, we don't ask the basic questions. We work backward from effects to causes, and are content with improvements and cures whose inner mechanisms we don't understand in detail. We ask ourselves questions that arise from our practice, we try to solve them by various approaches, simultaneous or consecutive, without any respect for accepted theories, and we aren't ashamed to admit it. If there is one area in which progress is made empirically, it is medicine. I hope it will always be so, and that the physician won't be prevented from trying to cure because the biologist hasn't yet elucidated everything. It was Einstein who pointed out that while the scientist explains what is, the engineer creates what has never been. We practicing doctors are content to be engineers, and we are resigned to not really knowing why we cure. And when the scientists fall ill, they come to see us.

There exists today a large and rapidly growing body of knowledge, a collection of "recipes" born of experimentation and observation, that enables us to cure cancers before we have been authorized to do so. The modern weapons of chemotherapy and immunotherapy, and our understanding of the optimum conditions of their use following surgery or radiotherapy, are products of that same empirical process by which the human mind has functioned ever since it was confronted with external reality. It is true that we can't yet cure all cancers, as knowledge of their ultimate causes will perhaps enable us to do one day. But the patients whom we do cure don't object—and their number is increasing regularly and significantly. It would increase much faster if applied, clinical research were given the serious support it deserves, instead of being treated in every program like the stepchild.

But as I have said, the results of treatment would be far more satisfactory even now if the knowledge we have already acquired were put into practice. That knowledge is not applied because for unconscious reasons most doctors join the basic scientists in believing that one doesn't fight cancer inch by inch, locked in dubious battle. Either one lays it low forever with a single blow of the scalpel, or else one is laid low by it. Hence the invincible skepticism that greets all the real but partial progress I have described. Hence the defeatism and the reluctance to organize the battle so as to give the patients every possible chance.

I don't know what disease will take the place of cancer and perform its function in the collective subconscious once cancer has given up all its secrets. Right now it is still cancer that is taboo. Every time oncologists try something beyond the conventional local treatments of surgery and radiation, other physicians, who themselves accept the challenge of other very serious diseases, accuse us of going too far. They base this accusation on the futility and harmfulness of general treatments, two notions I think I have refuted by many examples. I answer these practitioners with an accusation of my own. I consider that they are not doing enough in 1978 when they limit themselves to what we were able to do in 1970, and that it is their duty to keep themselves informed at first hand, from day to day, of the progress of medical oncology. I consider that when they choose to abstain from treatment, they are misinterpreting the will of the patients, who for their part, when they know the truth about their situation, choose to fight back and try their luck. Besides, patients know the truth infinitely more often than is generally believed. This means that in many cases the danger in the doctor's keeping silent and abstaining is not that the patient may be robbed of his death but that he may be robbed of his life.

If we censure those who stubbornly insist on treatment when it has no purpose, no real, appreciable chance of success, we must equally condemn those who stubbornly refuse to treat. It is easy to say to the relatives of an adult, "Let us bow to the inevitable; there's nothing more to be done." It was not so easy to say that to the mothers of young children with leukemia, who begged doctors to attempt the impossible and to take risks. That is one reason (there are others) why advances were made more rapidly in childhood leukemia than in other tumors. The hematologists really did attempt the impossible: the daring of the strategies they developed matched the dangers of the disease, and they obtained very encouraging results.

Cancer strikes oftener today than in the past. Its victims are chosen apparently at random, and they are younger all the time. The patients and their families are not resigned, and they are right. They don't turn up their noses at partial advances, because for the patient who benefits from them, they represent the difference between life and death.

It is true that we've made relatively little progress in treating cancers that are already disseminated or have recurred. In the vast majority of such cases, we haven't been able to cure but only to prolong survival. But having personally observed dozens of patients—and read of hundreds elsewhere—who have been saved contrary to all expectations, I've become convinced that I belong to the generation of doctors who will see the decisive breakthroughs in the treatment of these grave cases, and that our students will be the ones to carry the day.

I want to repeat that the great victories of recent years have been won by applying combined strategies to operable cases. We must immediately begin to consolidate our successes in this area with a proliferation of studies to determine precisely what is required for victory in each case. Already, with our present level of knowledge, we could greatly increase the number of patients who are cured, and cured under conditions that are entirely acceptable and always accepted by those who know what is at stake. People must be made aware of that fact. Conditions must be created so that the various combinations of treatments can be tested quickly and by the maximum number of competent physicians.

All this will doubtless upset many habits and create many unforeseen difficulties, bottlenecks, and conflicts. But that can't be helped. In the field of health, we are no more masters of our progress and its consequences than we are in other domains. Doctors aren't government officials or politicians, and it is not up to them to make the necessary adjustments in society. It is conceivable that under certain circumstances, geneticists might renounce studies that were potentially dangerous. But doctors can't deliberately restrain the progress of medicine in order not to create difficulties for society. The choice is whether to provide maximal medicine (multiply the number of centers for hemodialysis of kidney patients), minimal medicine (try merely to prevent great epidemics and control endemic diseases), or optimal medicine. Fortunately, it is not up to physicians to settle the argument. I conceive that my mission in society is to make improvements in the art of curing, and to place those improvements at the service of as many individuals as possible. What happens afterward is a matter of political choice and is therefore the responsibility of those who have a different sort of mission.

At the present time we are faced with many choices at once, and one sometimes feels that we have reached the limits of instability. What we need at this point is a cure for sick societies. Apparently, it does not yet exist. I only know, by analogy with my own work, that it will take engineers, not theoreticians, to find it.

Index

About the Author

Lucien Israël is head of the Hôpital Franco-Musulman in Bobigny, France, and is one of the few Europeans who is associated with the National Cancer Institute of the United States. He is also a member of the European Organization for Research on the Treatment of Cancer. Dr. Israël began his work as a pulmonary specialist, and his first cancer patients were suffering from lung cancer and had been given up by other doctors. As a result, he began to study all that was known about cancer and became a specialist in the field.